From Fear to Freedom:
A Workbook for Navigating Allergy Immunotherapy

Amanda R. DeSio Whitehouse, Ph.D.

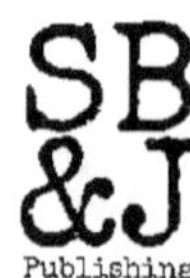
SB
&J
Publishing

One day you will tell your story of how you overcame what you went through,

and it will become someone else's survival guide.

-Brené Brown

Dedication

This book is for my boys, like everything else I do.

Being your Mom (Ama/Mama/Mother/TeacherMudder) has made me the best possible
version of myself. I can only hope that one day you'll be as thankful and proud as I am
of the way that our experiences together have shaped us as individuals and as a family.

I wish I could guarantee that you'd never have to go through hard things,
but I promise you that you'll never have to go through them without me by your side.

Table of Contents

Foreword

The food allergy field is in a remarkable moment. Treatment options have expanded dramatically in the past decade and protocols that would have seemed extraordinary not long ago are now available in clinics across the country. People who once had no options now have several. That is a profound shift for families who spent years believing there was no other way to live than avoid and carry epinephrine.

Yet the decision to pursue treatment, and the journey through it, remains one of the most psychologically complex experiences a food allergy patient or family can face. Here is something I have learned from navigating food allergy treatments with my own child, and from sitting with patients and families doing the same in my clinical work; You can read every study, consult every specialist, ask every question, and still arrive at the moment of decision carrying real uncertainty about whether you are doing the right thing.

Treatment decisions sit at the intersection of clinical data and gut feeling, of hope and fear, of what the research says and what it means to make a decision about your own body, or to be the parent who has to say yes. Or no. Or not yet. There is rarely a clear right answer, and there is almost always a significant emotional cost to whatever you choose. The anxiety. The ambivalence. The fear of the very thing that might help. The toll on the whole family, or the particular weight of navigating something this significant largely on your own as an adult. Allergists understand this. The psychosocial dimension of treatment is widely recognized as one of the most important and least resourced aspects of the patient journey. Not for lack of caring, but because the tools to address it haven't existed in any systematic way.

Dr. Amanda Whitehouse has spent years in that gap, as a psychologist and as a mother who has walked this road with her own son. This book is the result of that accumulated experience, and it arrives at exactly the right moment. What she has built here is something the field has needed: a comprehensive, warm, evidence-informed guide that takes patients and families through the full arc of the treatment journey, from first considerations through maintenance, without losing sight of the human being at the center of it.

Having worked in this space myself, I can speak to how much this resource adds to what has existed. Dr. Whitehouse has gone further into the emotional dimension of treatment than anything currently available, not just describing the journey but equipping people to navigate it. This book names what people are carrying, gives shape to what has felt shapeless, and offers tools for a journey that is, at its core, as much psychological as it is medical.

As a psychologist who has spent years working with food allergy patients and families, and as a food allergy parent myself, I can say with confidence that this resource will change how people experience treatment. Not by making it easier, exactly, but by making them feel less alone in it. Whatever brought you to this book, curiosity, fear, hope, exhaustion, or some complicated combination of all of them, you are in the right place. The journey ahead is real. So is the support you'll find here.

Elizabeth Hawkins, PhD, MPH
Licensed Psychologist
Co-Author of *Treating Food Allergies with Modern Medicine*
Founder, Food Allergy Hive

Getting Oriented

You probably picked up this book because something about the idea of a journey into allergy treatment resonates with you. Maybe you're ready to move forward. Maybe you're hesitant. Maybe you're exhausted, unsure if you even want to go anywhere, or unsure where "anywhere" might be.

I wrote this book and shared our own story in its pages because I understand how heavy and complex this process can feel. I know often it feels like you are expected to figure it out on your own. My hope is that these pages feel like company. That you feel supported as you think through your options, prepare for what might come, and move forward in a way that feels right for you.

I can't plan a trip for you, tell you exactly where you should go, or predict which path will be easiest, fastest, or most direct. What I can do is share my own journey and the journeys of others who have navigated their own paths. I can highlight some destinations you might consider, give you tips from experts, and help you notice the scenery along the way so you can find moments of ease, clarity, and even joy to stay focused on the entire journey, not just the destination.

Part Memoir, Part Guide, Part Workbook

This book is designed to meet you wherever you are on your journey. It blends memoir sections sharing real-life experiences from my own life and others' with reliable, evidence-informed information about food allergies, immunotherapy, and related strategies. It's also an interactive workbook, filled with prompts, charts, and exercises to help you actively engage with your own questions, concerns, and decisions. This unique combination allows you to learn, reflect, and plan, all in one place, so that the journey isn't something you have to navigate alone.

How It Started

Initially, I set out to record a season of my allergy anxiety podcast *Don't Feed the Fear* about immunotherapy. My goal was to walk listeners step-by-step through the growing number of treatment options from the earliest stages of decision-making to the daily realities of treatment if they chose that path. With each conversation, it became clear that the process was far more complex than a linear path. Every guest brought forward new insights, questions, and lived experiences that expanded the scope of what felt important to include.

Each guest shared an abundance of medical information or experience and acknowledged that understanding of and support for the mental health aspect is essential. I realized that what was still missing was guidance on how to navigate the social and emotional dimensions of these decisions: the fear, the uncertainty, the family dynamics, and the internal conflicts that often accompany them. This workbook was created to help fill that space.

It is designed to complement medical guidance by helping you integrate the non-medical factors that are just as critical in making informed, sustainable decisions. Throughout these pages, you'll find reflections and excerpts inspired by conversations with clinicians and patient advocates walking through all angles of these decisions. I hope it will feel like a guided conversation that supports you in making decisions that are not only medically sound, but emotionally and practically aligned with your own life.

Stories, Facts, and Tools: Why They Belong Together

If you are walking this path holding fear and hope in the same breath, learning a language you never wanted to speak, trying to be brave while your nervous system is on high alert, I want you to know from your first step that you are not alone. I'm sharing our story so you'll know I truly understand, and so you can learn from both my experiences and the knowledge I've gained from clients and the experts I've been fortunate to connect with along the way.

While reliving our story scrolling through photos, confirming dates, reviewing appointment notes and bloodwork results, what stood out most was my son's bravery and maturity. He handled something extraordinarily complex with grace that I couldn't fully appreciate at the time. Writing this book became an unexpected part of my own integration process.

Narrative therapy is based on the idea that the stories we tell about our lives shape how we understand ourselves. Writing allows us to gently take those experiences out of the background and place them somewhere we can see them, organize them, and relate to them differently. That's what this book has been for me. And as you move through these pages, I hope that's what it will help you do, too.

Writing about emotions has been shown to reduce activation in the brain's threat-detection system. When feelings stay unspoken and unprocessed, the brain often treats them as unresolved danger, requiring ongoing vigilance and mental energy. Writing gives those experiences somewhere to go.

Compared to talking, writing engages a wider network of brain regions involved in memory, meaning-making, and integration. It helps shift experiences out of short-term, emotionally charged storage and into long-term memory, where they can be "filed away" rather than constantly revisited.

When we put words to what we feel, we also activate the prefrontal cortex, the part of the brain responsible for reasoning, planning, and intentional decision-making. This doesn't erase emotion, but it creates space around it that can allow us to observe instead of react, and choose how to respond, and when not to.

Writing also reduces rumination. Instead of cycling through the same thoughts internally, you create distance from them on the page. That distance allows perspective, clarity, and often compassion to emerge naturally.

Even when you aren't writing directly about emotions, the act of writing itself is regulating. Making a list, outlining a plan, or jotting down observations engages brain regions involved in organization and problem-solving. This can help shift you out of emotional overload and into a more grounded, focused state.

That's why this book includes worksheets, prompts, and spaces for you to write. Don't think of it as busywork or something to be done "right." The act of writing your responses is therapeutic.

I strongly encourage you to write by hand when possible. Writing physically rather than just reading, typing, or thinking requires coordination between cognitive and motor systems in the brain. This naturally slows the process down, giving your nervous system more time to process information and assign meaning. Even brief notes can be effective. Write pages if you like, or jot down a few words, a sentence, or a list. What matters is that you give your story somewhere to land.

My hope is that as you read others' experiences alongside your own reflections, you'll begin to see your story with more clarity and less isolation. May this workbook help you see where fear has been gripping the steering wheel, where your nervous system has been running in overdrive, and where resilience has been quietly riding shotgun all along.

How to Use This Book

This book is written for you as an adult, whether patient or parent, to support you in more than one way. Each section will include clear information from reliable and trusted sources to help you understand the topic. Personal stories throughout reflect the emotional experience of that topic. Finally, you'll be invited to integrate the new information with your own emotions and experience by engaging in the worksheets and activities. Some activities are designed for you to reflect and explore on your own as a patient or parent. Others are meant to be shared with a child to support their understanding, growth, and participation in their own journey.

To make it easier to move between these different kinds of reading, you'll see the following icons throughout the book. Switching between learning, feeling, and doing can be demanding, so these icons provide a visual cue that helps you know what kind of attention the next section is asking for.

The Four Icons You'll See

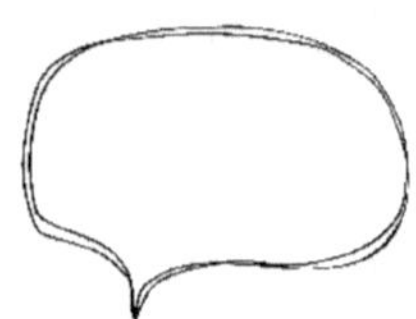

Memoirs & Lived Experiences

When you see the speech bubble, the section shares a personal story, reflection, or vignette. These moments are here to help you feel less alone, to normalize the emotional side of this process, and to offer connection and meaning rather than instruction.

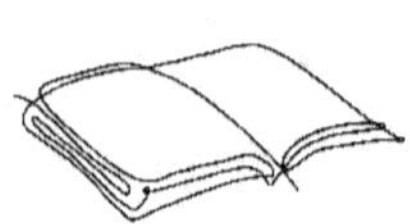

Learning & Understanding

When you see the open book icon, the section is informational. These sections explain medical concepts, nervous system science, and treatment details. You can read these sections at your own pace, revisit them as needed, and come back to them as reference material.

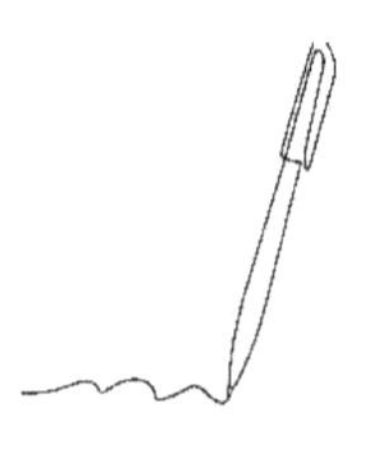

Your Turn: Practice & Reflection

When you see the pen icon, the book is inviting you to participate. These sections include worksheets, reflection prompts, and activities you can do on your own or with your child. You don't need to complete every activity. Use what feels supportive and skip what doesn't.

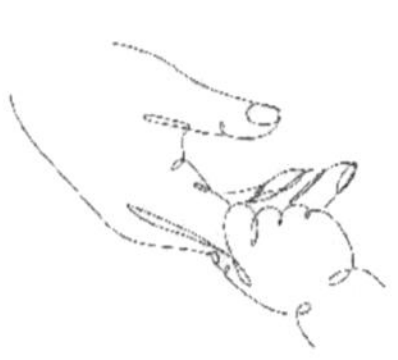

Involving your Child

You'll see this icon on child-facing activities meant to be facilitated by an adult. They are designed to be adaptable across a wide range of ages and developmental levels. These exercises are intended to be completed together with your child, with you guiding, narrating, and regulating alongside them.

The children's activity pages are not intended to be handed to children to complete on their own. Even if something seems simplistic for your child's age, remember that emotional maturity regarding stressful topics often differs from intelligence, and simplicity around challenging topics can feel comforting. Your active involvement signals to your child that this work isn't "for little kids," it is support for anyone going through this process. Remember that the goal for these activities is shared experience and emotional safety. Keep a collection of colorful papers, fun markers or crayons, and stickers on hand to make these activities more engaging. Most of these activities will be completed on separate paper, not directly in this workbook.

Some older teens may benefit from reading selected sections of the book or completing certain adult worksheets *together with their parent or caregiver.* Even so, this book is not meant to be handed over to them to read alone. Even mature, thoughtful, or highly intelligent children can get overwhelmed with content that can feel heavy, technical, or emotionally loaded. This topic is overwhelming enough for us as adults.

This collaborative, parent-led approach is intentional and crucial. Nervous system regulation is most effectively supported by a safe, trusted adult. By making togetherness explicit rather than assuming independence, we help children feel safer, more contained, and more supported as they navigate a challenging medical journey.

Types of Activities

Throughout this workbook, you will encounter a variety of activities and exercises designed to support both the practical and emotional aspects of navigating food allergy treatment decisions. These exercises draw from well-established approaches within psychology and behavioral health, each offering different tools for understanding thoughts, emotions, behaviors, and the nervous system's response to stress. The descriptions below briefly explain the general categories of psychological approaches represented in the workbook. These are shared to help you to better understand the intention behind each exercise and explore the approaches that resonate most with you/your child.

Cognitive Behavioral Therapy (CBT)*:* Helps identify and challenge unhelpful thoughts, reduce anxiety, and develop practical coping strategies. CBT helps individuals identify, challenge, and replace thoughts, beliefs, and behavior patterns that reinforce anxiety, avoidance, or distress.

Acceptance and Commitment Therapy (ACT): A type of CBT that focuses on psychological flexibility and values-driven action.

Exposure-Based Strategies: Another CBT approach that supports gradually confronting fears or triggers in a safe, structured way to build confidence and tolerance.

Nervous System Regulation Practices: Techniques to calm the body and mind, reduce hyperarousal, and build resilience in stressful situations. These approaches focus on shifting out of survival states (fight, flight, freeze) into a more regulated state of safety and connection. This includes tools for breath, movement, and vocalization. This also includes the crucial strategy of co-regulation, where a caregiver uses calm presence, empathy, and nervous system regulation to help a child return to a regulated state.

Mindfulness and Somatic Awareness: Practices that increase awareness of bodily sensations, emotions, and thoughts without judgment. Mindfulness teaches present-moment awareness without judgment.

Trauma-Informed Practices: These practices acknowledge the impact of trauma on development and behavior, and prioritize safety, trust, and empowerment. Focus is on emotional safety and reducing re-traumatization.

Narrative Reflection/Journaling/Expressive Arts: Encourages exploring personal stories and experiences, making sense of challenges, and fostering insight. These interventions allow us to process experiences creatively and support emotional processing when verbal expression may be difficult.

Self-Compassion Practices: Building kindness toward oneself, especially in the face of setbacks, mistakes, or medical challenges.

Values Clarification/Motivation Work: Identifying what matters most to you and using those values to guide decisions and actions. These tools help you identify your "why," the values that motivate you to persevere through treatment. This includes goal-setting and anchoring routines in meaningful reasons for continuing.

Problem-Solving and Decision-Making Skills: Practical tools for weighing options, setting priorities, and planning steps forward.

Psychoeducation: Understanding the science behind allergies, treatment options, and emotional responses to empower informed choices.

Disclaimer

This workbook is designed to provide education, tools, and emotional support to families navigating immunotherapy or other treatments for food allergies. It is based on evidence-informed approaches with the goal of supporting emotional well-being during the treatment process. Sharing a resource does not imply an approval, endorsement, or any sort of affiliation with that resource or its creators.

Not Medical Advice

The content in this workbook is not intended to provide medical advice, diagnosis, or treatment. It does not replace professional medical guidance from your allergist or any other healthcare provider. In-depth medical explanations are beyond the scope of this book. Always consult your medical team before making any changes to your treatment/allergy action plan. If you have questions or concerns about symptoms, reactions, or protocols related to immunotherapy or any treatment, speak directly with your allergist or medical provider. *Do not attempt any of these treatments without individualized medical guidance from your physician or other healthcare provider.*

The information in this book comes from these carefully selected sources:

• Conversations with leading physicians and researchers who joined me to share their expertise and insights on the *Don't Feed The Fear* podcast, summarized in this book with their permission/review
• Peer-reviewed research studies
• Personal experiences shared with permission

The medical content in this book has been reviewed for accuracy by allergist/immunologist Dr. Allison Freeman. Mental health content has been reviewed for accuracy by psychologist Dr. Elizabeth Hawkins. In addition, sections featuring insights or content drawn from podcast interviews with physician guests have been reviewed by those individuals for accuracy and approval.

For a deeper understanding of the medical topics discussed, the following excellent books written by food allergy experts are helpful resources:

> *The End of Food Allergy* by Dr. Kari Nadeau
> *The Complete Guide to Food Allergies in Adults and Children* by Dr. Scott Sicherer
> *Food Without Fear* by Dr. Ruchi Gupta
> *All About Allergies* by Dr. Zachary Rubin

Not a Substitute for Mental Health Treatment

While the exercises and tools provided in this workbook may support emotional regulation and resilience, they are not a substitute for therapy or psychological diagnosis. You are strongly encouraged to seek help from a licensed mental health professional if you or your child are experiencing:

- Ongoing or escalating anxiety that interferes with daily functioning
- Panic attacks or extreme fear regarding immunotherapy doses
- Depression, withdrawal, hopelessness, thoughts of harming self/others

- Changes in sleep, appetite, weight/clothing size
- Difficulty coping despite use of supportive tools and strategies
- Trauma symptoms related to past allergic reactions or medical care
- Avoidance of food, school, professional, or social activities

Sensitive Content Warning

This workbook contains discussion of severe allergic reactions, emergency responses, injections/needles, and other sensitive topics. Readers with a history of anxiety, trauma, or heightened emotional sensitivity to these subjects are encouraged to engage with the material gradually and with appropriate support if needed.

Part I:
Introduction

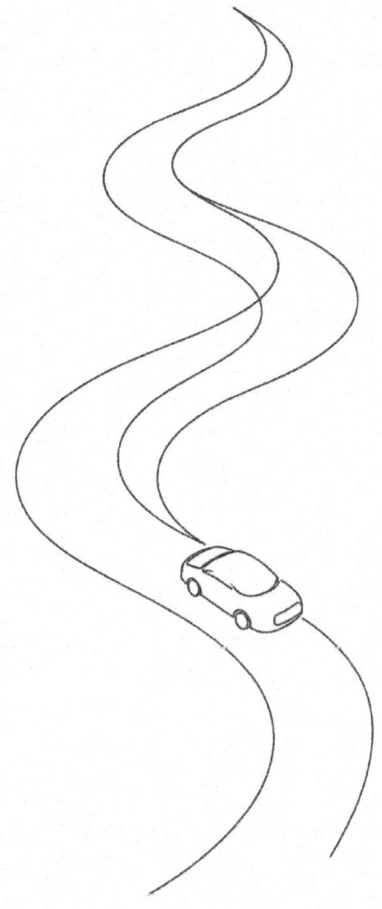

Do not expect to find yourself
using someone else's map.

— Leigh Standley

When my son was first diagnosed with food allergies at 16 months old, I could not accept being told that there was nothing we could do but avoid his allergens (even though the full list of those was still unclear) and carry epinephrine. I turned to my favorite and most reliable coping skill: I started reading everything I could find.

I searched medical journals, followed pioneering researchers like they were rock stars, and asked questions. I asked so many questions that I was kicked out of more than one allergist's office for asking about treatments I learned about in peer-reviewed articles. I felt motivated, determined, and incredibly alone.

I never want another parent to feel the way I did during those early years as an allergy parent. I was desperate for information and confident that there must be some treatment available or being developed that could help my son. I did not write this book to convince you to begin immunotherapy or biologic medications. I wrote it so you don't have to navigate this alone, and maybe also for the version of myself who needed it almost fourteen years ago.

Those early years of my son's food allergies were marked by constant alertness and a deep sense of unpredictability. Our days were filled with mystery reactions that we were repeatedly told were impossible but kept happening anyway. He experienced anaphylaxis after a dog licked him, despite there being no allergen in the dog's food. He reacted at a baseball game where peanuts were present in the air despite never being out of my arms, eating anything, or touching any surfaces. He had an anaphylactic reaction to blowing bubbles, which I later learned contained peanut oil. He developed full body hives from library books, the belt at the grocery store checkout, soap in public bathrooms, and the hickory nuts that fell in our own yard. Each experience reinforced the same message in my body, over and over again: the world was unpredictable and safety required constant vigilance.

At the time, I understood trauma from a scientific and clinical lens. Living through these experiences transformed that understanding completely. Repeated reactions, constant uncertainty, and the ongoing awareness of stories about children who had died from food allergy reactions created a cumulative impact that was not acknowledged, socially or medically. What others framed as unwarranted anxiety was, in reality, a nervous system shaped by repeated experiences of threat. That was true not only for my child, but for me as a parent witnessing it again and again.

I knew that this was not a healthy way for either of us to live, regardless of how carefully I tried to manage it. Even if I could keep him physically safe, the social and emotional cost was becoming too high. I could feel it in my own body as much as I could see it in his world shrinking. The cost of those years was not always visible to others, though some thought I was "high strung" and "controlling." I realize that their perceptions were likely based on a lack of understanding of how dangerous food allergies can be, and how food allergies impact all areas of life. I tried to be present and stay calm outwardly, but looking back I see how often my mind was elsewhere: scanning, planning, anticipating the next possible risk. I missed moments I can never get back, because I was always bracing. I wanted to create a calm, gentle upbringing for my children, so I worked hard to appear steady on the outside while my body was carrying a very different experience on the inside. I struggled to sleep and eat, my nervous system rarely settled, and the toll on my body would not fully become clear until years later, after my son reached maintenance for all his food allergens.

As I charged ahead into our long and winding immunotherapy journey, it changed us and our lives in ways that I couldn't have anticipated. I found myself wanting to share that reality with families who were still standing at the beginning, unsure whether they could or should make it through. Immunotherapy is not the right choice for every patient or family. But in my work as a psychologist, I have seen many people avoid treatment because their anxiety and trauma made it feel overwhelming or impossible, not because it was medically inappropriate for them. I have also seen people who initially resisted the idea out of fear go on to benefit deeply when they had the right information and support to help them navigate the process.

The skills I'd developed as my son's advocate in the grocery store and on the playground were very useful when immunotherapy began. There were many moments when navigating treatment felt overwhelming and even impossible. There were times I wanted to give up and times I worried that we had made the wrong decision. However, my son was so incredibly sensitive and reactive to his allergens that careful avoidance was not keeping him physically or emotionally safe. Treatment seemed like the only option, regardless of how challenging, time-consuming, and expensive it might be. I don't share this to be dramatic or to scare anyone, but because patients and families managing highly reactive allergies like my son's are often the most afraid to pursue treatment. Yet they are also the ones whose lives are most significantly impacted by fear and restriction. They are also the ones who need the most support to see the process through in a way that feels safe and sustainable.

I managed these challenges in my own home with my family while having the privilege of working as a psychologist with my clients who are also navigating the complex emotional landscape of food allergies. Every session and conversation has deepened my understanding of what it is like to live with these daily challenges. All of the experience I have gathered, directly and vicariously, is reflected in this book.

This book is for you if you are standing at that edge, weighing difficult decisions while your nervous system is already stretched thin. It is for you if you are curious, hopeful, and afraid. It is for you if you are holding everything together on the outside while feeling perpetually vigilant inside. And it is for you if you want to make decisions that combine evidence-based information, mental clarity, emotional support, and compassion for your child or yourself, rather than from fear alone.

Introductory Activity: A Compassionate Letter to Yourself

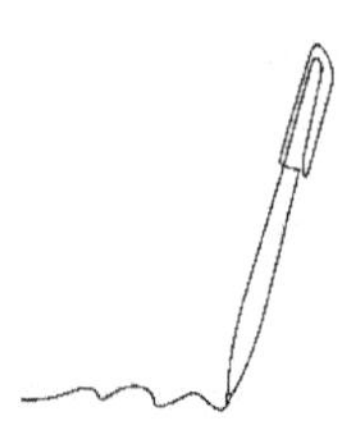

If you are reading this book, it is likely because something about allergy management and/or the possibility of seeking treatment already feels heavy. You may be carrying confusion, fear, grief, exhaustion, guilt, hope, or a complicated mix of it all. You may be eager to "get to the helpful parts," to gather information, to feel more prepared or more in control. That impulse makes sense. You're seeking clarity.

But the goal of this book isn't just to choose something. It's to get your mind and body in sync to make a grounded and informed decision. When we push forward without first acknowledging what we're already holding, our nervous systems often stay in a guarded state, absorbing information intellectually while remaining emotionally braced. When that happens, even good information can feel overwhelming. There's a good chance that's the state you're already in. This brief exercise is meant to help your body and brain feel safe and connected enough to receive what comes next.

Research shows that compassionate, reflective writing can reduce shame, soften self-criticism, and increase emotional regulation. When we write from a place of kindness toward ourselves, even briefly, we engage the parts of the brain involved in perspective-taking, meaning-making, and intentional decision-making. This creates a steadier internal foundation for learning, planning, and problem-solving (Swee, Klein, Murray, & Heimberg, 2023).

Just as importantly, this exercise establishes how I hope you will and will not use this book. I hope you *won't* view it as a checklist, a measure of how "right" your decisions are, or another list of things you "should" be doing. Instead, please utilize this exercise to move forward from a place of connection and self-awareness, meeting yourself wherever you are in this moment. You can note where you wish you were and where you think you should be, while gently acknowledging that in this moment you are *here*. From that place, everything else in this book becomes more accessible. The tools land more gently, the information feels less threatening, and the exercises become supportive rather than demanding.

Taking a few minutes to write this letter helps set the tone for learning and work ahead that is rooted in compassion, curiosity, and steadiness rather than fear or urgency. It gives your story and your nervous system a place to begin.

Instructions

Write a letter to yourself honestly, openly, and without judgment. You might include:

1. How you are feeling right now about your allergies, treatments, or the journey ahead
2. Any hopes, fears, or uncertainties you have
3. Why you are reading this book, and what you want to learn more about or better understand
4. What you want to remember as you move forward

Dear Me,

____

____

____

____

____

____

____

____

____

____

____

____

____

____

____

When you are done, close the book, take a breath, and sit with whatever comes up for a moment.

Choice, Control, and the Weight of Decision-Making

 For many years, the standard message given to individuals and families managing food allergies was simple and absolute: avoid the allergen and carry epinephrine. There was clarity in that guidance, but there was also a profound absence of choice. There were no meaningful alternatives to consider, no decisions to weigh, and very little sense of control over the trajectory of life with food allergies.

Today, that landscape has changed. Families are now presented with multiple options, including oral immunotherapy (OIT), sublingual immunotherapy (SLIT), the Tolerance Induction Program (TIP), biologic medications, and even more emerging approaches. This expansion is both hopeful and, for many, deeply overwhelming.

To understand why, it is helpful to look at what psychological research tells us about choice.

Why Choice Matters

Decades of research have shown that having choice is not just a practical benefit, but a psychological one. The ability to make decisions is closely tied to autonomy, motivation, and well-being. When individuals are given choices, they tend to feel more engaged, more capable, and more satisfied with outcomes, even when the options themselves are relatively small or incidental.

Research has demonstrated that even minor opportunities for choice can significantly improve psychological and physical well-being. Simple choices about our experiences are connected to improved mood, increased engagement, and better health outcomes compared to those who were not given these choices (Langer & Rodin, 1976). Individuals who are allowed to choose aspects of their experience demonstrate greater motivation, persistence, and performance (Cordova & Lepper, 1996).

These findings are so consistent that the ability to make meaningful choices is widely considered a fundamental psychological need (Deci & Ryan, 1985). When that need is supported, individuals are more likely to experience a sense of agency and well-being.

In the context of food allergies, this shift from having no options to having multiple options can be profoundly meaningful. Even for families who ultimately decide not to pursue a specific treatment, the ability to consider and evaluate those options can foster a greater sense of control and confidence.

When More Choice Becomes Overwhelming

At the same time, more choice is not always better. Psychological research has also shown that when the number or complexity of options exceeds what a person can reasonably process, decision-making can become more difficult and less satisfying. This phenomenon is often referred to as choice overload (Iyengar & Lepper, 2000; Misuraca et al., 2024).

When individuals are presented with too many options, several patterns tend to emerge. Decision-making may be delayed or avoided altogether. Confidence in the chosen option may decrease. Satisfaction after making a decision may be lower. Individuals may also experience increased regret or second-guessing. Our cognitive systems have limits, and when we are asked to weigh multiple options with many variables, risks, and uncertainties, especially in emotionally significant contexts, the process can become mentally and emotionally taxing (Misuraca et al., 2024).

In the case of food allergy treatment, these decisions are rarely simple. They often involve weighing safety, quality of life, time commitment, financial cost, complex medical concepts, potential risks, personal values, and the needs of multiple family members. The stakes feel high because they *are* high. It is not surprising that many feel overwhelmed when navigating these choices.

Holding Both Sides: Empowerment and Overwhelm

What this means in practice is that the current moment in food allergy care holds two truths. The first is that having options is a meaningful and positive shift that can increase a sense of agency and open doors to improved safety and quality of life. The second truth is that these options can introduce uncertainty, increase pressure to make the "right" decision, and create space for doubt, guilt, and second-guessing.

Finding Your Place Within the Options

This workbook is designed with these realities in mind. It is not meant to present every possible option in a way that requires you to evaluate them all at once. Instead, it is meant to help you organize, reflect, and move through decisions at a pace and depth that feels manageable.

The act of thoughtfully considering options, clarifying your values, and understanding what is available can improve confidence and reduce distress, regardless of the final decision (Misuraca et al., 2024). In other words, engaging with the process itself has value.

Whether you move toward a specific treatment, decide to wait, or choose to continue with your current approach, the goal is the same: to arrive at a decision that feels informed, aligned, and steady enough to carry forward.

This Book Is a Travel Guide, Not a Map

As you move through this book, it may help to think of this process as a journey that you're considering taking. For many, food allergy life has already felt like a long journey including moments of fear, learning, adjustment, and hopefully growth. Deciding whether to pursue immunotherapy, and what that might look like for you or your child, is not a simple yes or no decision. It is a path that unfolds over time, and this is a journey that you get to choose whether or not to take.

Like any journey, there may be stretches that feel clear and steady, and others that feel uncertain or difficult to navigate. There may be moments where you move forward with confidence, and others where you pause, question, or change direction. You may take a path that looks very different from someone else's, and that does not mean you are doing it wrong.

This book will not tell you which direction to go or whether to go anywhere at all. It is a travel guide, not a map. You do not have to visit every site or use every resource inside it. You are not meant to read it front to back. You are not required to complete every worksheet. You are not falling behind if you skip exercises that don't feel helpful or apply to you. At some points you may benefit from deep reflection, and other times you may only need quick reference and clarity. The pages, prompts, and decision tools are not a checklist. It is a collection of options that may or may not feel supportive.

I included a wide range of frameworks, worksheets, and reflection tools because everyone enters this journey from their own starting point. Some are newly diagnosed and overwhelmed. Some are considering immunotherapy. Some are steady in avoidance but struggling psychologically. Some are ready to reassess and change paths.

If food allergy treatment were a highway leading to one destination with clear exits and predictable traffic, you wouldn't need this book. Someone would simply hand you a map, highlight the fastest route, and send you on your way. In fact, for years that's what our doctors did: avoid the allergens and carry epinephrine.

Managing food allergies today is much more like planning your own trip. There are multiple possible destinations. There are scenic paths and direct routes. There are detours, road closures, weather shifts, and moments when you pull over to regroup. And perhaps most importantly, there isn't one "correct" destination or a definitive way to get there.

That is why this book is not a map, but a travel guide that describes the terrain, highlights and landmarks. It explains what different regions are like and what travelers might encounter there. It helps you understand what to expect so that when you make your decisions, you do so with more clarity than before, even though it can't predict all the factors you'll encounter.

Sometimes, a travel guide serves another equally important purpose: it helps you decide not to take the trip. You may read these pages and realize that this is a journey that, for now or for the foreseeable future, is not for you. You may determine that the cost in time, money, energy, or emotional strain outweighs the benefits for you in this season. If this book helps you come to that conclusion before investing significant resources into a path that doesn't align with your goals or capacity, hopefully you'll consider that a success.

Every intentional journey includes reassessment. You might begin with the goal of maintaining confident avoidance and later decide you want to increase protection. You might consider oral immunotherapy and realize that it is the wrong season. You might move forward enthusiastically and later decide to pause. Changing course is part of careful navigation, so think of yourself as a traveler.

This is your journey.

Part II:
Understanding The Journey

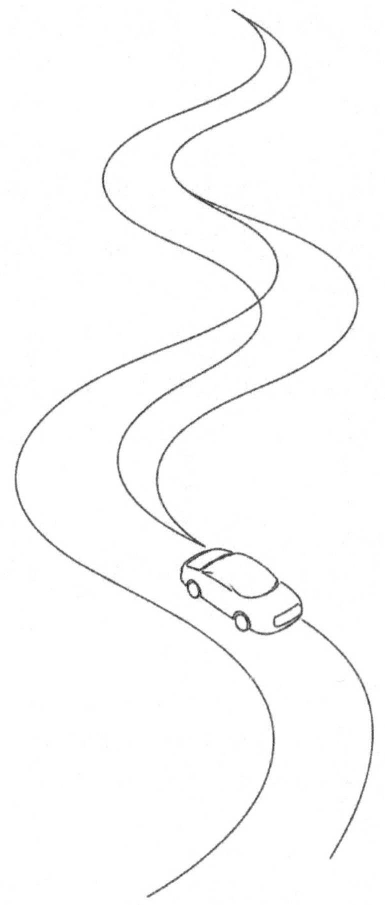

Problem talk creates problems.
Solution talk creates solutions.

— Steve de Shazer

Chapter 1:
Understanding Immunotherapy Options

Food allergy immunotherapy is a treatment approach designed to change how the immune system responds to specific allergens. The idea is simple, and the process is precise: Allergists give the body a tiny amount of the allergen, carefully measured so it does not trigger a dangerous reaction, and then gradually increase the dose over time.

This "training" allows the immune system to learn that the allergen is not a threat. Instead, it is a way to increase tolerance, decrease the severity of reactions if they occur, and reduce the constant anxiety and hyper-vigilance that often accompany living with food allergies.

Your nervous system and immune system are deeply connected. Imagine that your body has a built-in alarm system that is very sensitive to allergens. In someone with a food allergy, even a small amount of a particular food can trigger a severe reaction. Immunotherapy works by giving the body safe experiences with the allergen, repeatedly and gradually. Each exposure is like telling the body, "This is okay. You are safe." Over time, this repeated learning helps the body respond with calm instead of alarm.

Paths Forward

All forms of immunotherapy gradually introduce the immune system to an allergen in a controlled, medically supervised way to build tolerance over time. Each approach differs in important ways, but this shared concept can make the process feel more understandable as you learn about newer or less familiar options.

- *Oral Immunotherapy (OIT):* Small doses of the allergen are taken by mouth and gradually increased over time.
- *Tolerance Induction Program (TIP):* Uses "biosimilar" (structurally similar) proteins from other foods to train the immune system safely before introducing the actual allergen gradually into the diet.
- *Sublingual Immunotherapy (SLIT):* The allergen is placed under the tongue in small, controlled doses. SLIT is available for both environmental and food allergies.
- *Subcutaneous Immunotherapy (SCIT):* "Allergy shots" deliver small doses of the allergen over time. SCIT is an option for environmental allergies only, not food allergies.
- *Biologic medications* are another available treatment that target the immune system, but they do not retrain it to tolerate the allergens. These medications are delivered via injection and target specific immune receptors to reduce specific allergic conditions. They can be used alone or in combination with other immunotherapy approaches.

Each of these options will be explained in more detail so you can better understand how they work and what the experience may look like for patients. Several other promising immunotherapy options being developed or in research that may be available soon will also be discussed. Hopefully, this book will require frequent updates to cover the many new exciting choices becoming available.

Oral Immunotherapy

Oral immunotherapy (OIT), is currently the most widely studied, best understood, and most accessible treatment for food allergies. As the name suggests, OIT involves daily oral ingestion of gradually increasing amounts of a specific food allergen with the goal of retraining the immune system to tolerate it without reaction. OIT has been shown to be effective in increasing reaction thresholds, allowing many individuals to safely tolerate larger amounts of their allergen. It is considered safe when conducted under medical supervision, though reactions can occur during treatment (Nurmatov et al., 2014).

Despite its safety, the idea of intentionally eating a food that has caused an allergic reaction or has been avoided as potentially life-threatening can feel overwhelming or even unthinkable for many patients and parents. The sections that follow will first build a clear understanding of what OIT is and how it works, and then address the emotional and psychological experiences that can arise throughout the process.

Careful Calculation

OIT begins with microscopic amounts of the food protein a person is allergic to. These doses are carefully calculated and measured to be below the individual's threshold of reactivity. In other words, treatment begins below the level that would typically trigger symptoms, according to Dr. Doug Jones in episode 78 of the *Don't Feed the* Fear podcast (Whitehouse & Jones, 2026). Dr. Jones is a board-certified allergist and immunologist known for his pioneering work in oral immunotherapy (OIT) in his clinical practice, and for his widely followed platform @drdougjones, where he helps families understand how to think about risk, predictability, and control in real-world food allergy management. He is the co-founder and president of the Food Allergy Support Team (FAST), a nonprofit dedicated to supporting allergists, staff, and patients with immunotherapy.

After initial OIT dosing, the immune system is gradually guided to tolerate larger and larger amounts of the food through precise timing, structured dosing intervals, and medical oversight. The updosing process is done deliberately and precisely. The goal is to raise the threshold of tolerance with repeated safe exposures over time. If a person previously reacted to a crumb, over time they may tolerate a bite or even a full serving. For some, the destination is what is sometimes called "free eating," meaning they can consume that food without restriction. For others, the goal is simply protection from accidental exposures. OIT can and should be individualized to meet the patient's individual medical and social/emotional needs.

OIT can be completed for a single food or multiple allergens. Upon reaching the desired dose(s), which varies depending on the patient and their goals, a "maintenance" dose is maintained moving forward. For some, this may be incorporating the food into the diet regularly, and for others this is a measured dose that is consistently consumed.

Gaining Perspective on Risk
For many families, the idea of intentionally ingesting an allergen feels unthinkable. Fear is understandable, and food allergy reactions can cause trauma that persists long after the reaction. Dr. Jones acknowledged

this fear directly. He explained that many clinicians felt dissatisfied with offering only hope and vigilance. OIT emerged not as a reckless experiment, but as a structured, evidence-based option to increase safety.

He offered a metaphor that powerfully offers perspective on risk in immunotherapy: OIT is like flying on an airplane (Whitehouse & Jones, 2026). Flying can feel frightening and people imagine worst-case scenarios like turbulence, storms, and mechanical failure. Yet before any plane leaves the ground, there are preflight checks. The aircraft is inspected, the crew reviews procedures, the weather is assessed, flight paths are planned, and contingencies are prepared for. Safety is not assumed, it is engineered.

OIT follows the same principle. Before each dose, patients are taught to complete what Dr. Jones calls "pre-dose checks." Is the patient healthy today? Is asthma controlled? Has there been recent illness? Are there any signs that the body is already under stress? These questions assess and reduce turbulence. Just as a pilot would not fly into a storm without preparation, OIT is not advanced blindly. Doses are given at predictable times, in controlled settings, with clear instructions in place.

Turbulence does not mean disaster. If a plane encounters rough air, the pilot can change altitude, adjust speed, and reroute. In OIT, if a patient experiences symptoms, the dose can be adjusted, the schedule can be slowed, and supportive medications can be used. The process is dynamic and responsive.

Dr. Jones often reminds families that statistically, flying is safer than driving. In the same way, he argues that structured immunotherapy may carry less risk than a lifetime of unpredictable accidental exposures. A reaction at a birthday party or restaurant can happen without warning. A reaction during OIT, if it occurs, happens within a system designed to anticipate and manage it (Whitehouse & Jones, 2026).

That does not mean risk disappears. Reactions can happen and epinephrine is needed for a small portion of people doing OIT. Estimates of the percentage of patients experiencing anaphylaxis requiring epinephrine during the first year of treatment vary widely. They occur most often in the up-dosing phase and risk decreases over time. Severe anaphylaxis is rare and more likely to occur in milk OIT and for those with asthma (Patel, Vazquez-Ortiz, & Turner, 2019). A detailed review of the risk of anaphylaxis during OIT is beyond the scope of this book, and should be discussed with your doctor based on your individual risk factors.

Fear is magnified by misinformation. The understanding that doses start below reaction thresholds and are advanced with caution can help to shift anxiety from catastrophic imagination to informed preparation.

Candidates for OIT

There are some temporary barriers to starting OIT, according to Dr. Jones (Whitehouse & Jones, 2026). Uncontrolled asthma, poorly managed eczema, active hives, or severe unmanaged anxiety may increase risk or complicate the OIT process. Instead of seeing these as permanent disqualifications, they can be considered signals to stabilize before takeoff. Once underlying conditions are controlled, most individuals can be candidates.

Even conditions once considered prohibitive, such as eosinophilic esophagitis (EoE), are now viewed with more nuance. With careful monitoring and newer medical therapies available, many patients with EoE can safely participate in immunotherapy. EoE warrants its own more detailed discussion in a later chapter of this workbook, but overall it is important to understand that OIT treatment is evolving and experience and collaboration among allergists have refined protocols and improved safety.

Ultimately, OIT is not about forcing anyone to eat a food they dislike or fear. Some patients achieve free eating and choose not to consume the food regularly. They simply value the increased safety and protection from accidents. Each choice is valid, and each patient can choose their own destination. Flying is not mandatory, but for those who choose to board the plane, knowing that the aircraft has been inspected, the route planned, and the crew trained can make all the difference.

Dosing Commitments and Safety Precautions

When considering OIT, it is important to have a realistic understanding of the day-to-day commitments involved. While protocols vary by provider and treatment type, most approaches to immunotherapy include a set of guidelines designed to support safety and consistency.

This content is not a substitute for medical advice. Your allergist or treatment team will provide specific instructions tailored to you or your child. The goal here is to help you understand the general structure and expectations so you can make an informed decision and feel prepared for what participation may involve.

Because OIT involves repeated, controlled exposure to an allergen, safety protocols are essential to minimize the risk of reactions and ensure the best possible outcomes. Numerous peer-reviewed studies and clinical guidelines emphasize important precautions and safety protocols (Mack et al., 2024; Nurmatov et al., 2014).

Important note: Each allergist or treatment center may use specific protocols that differ in details such as dosing schedules, up-dose increments, and activity restrictions. Always follow the individualized plan provided by your care team and ask questions if anything is unclear.

General safety elements commonly recommended in clinical practice and described in peer-reviewed OIT literature include:

Medication Management
Patients must have epinephrine readily available and know how and when to use it.

Epinephrine & Emergency Plan
A clear, written emergency action plan should be reviewed and practiced with caregivers. Knowing when and how to use epinephrine is an essential part of safety.

Daily Dosing Routine
OIT requires consistent daily ingestion of the prescribed dose of allergen to maintain desensitization. Missing doses or inconsistent timing can reduce effectiveness and increase risk.

Take Doses with Food
Doses are typically taken on a full stomach, often one that includes carbohydrates. Eating prior to dosing can help reduce gastrointestinal discomfort and may lower the risk of systemic reactions.

Timing of Physical Activity
Many protocols recommend avoiding strenuous exercise or intense physical activity for approximately 2 hours after dosing, because increased exertion can trigger reactions. Exercise avoidance for a shorter period prior to dosing may also be recommended. This is commonly described as one of the most difficult requirements of OIT for children to adhere to.

Temperature
Avoiding activities that raise body temperature around the time of dosing (e.g., hot showers, baths, saunas) is recommended as this may increase the likelihood of symptoms.

NSAID Avoidance
Nonsteroidal anti-inflammatory drugs (NSAIDs, such as ibuprofen) may increase reaction risk and are often avoided around dosing unless specifically approved by the provider.

Illness Protocols
If the participant has a fever, active infection, vomiting, or significant fatigue, the allergist may recommend holding or reducing the dose until recovery to prevent heightened sensitivity during illness.

Menstruation
Females undergoing oral immunotherapy (OIT) typically do not need to stop dosing during menstruation, but some doctors may recommend lowering the dose during the first few days of the cycle. Hormonal changes during this time can impact dose tolerance.

Additional important factors to discuss with your provider include active infection, uncontrolled allergic disease, asthma exacerbation, tiredness or sleep deprivation, dental work or oral trauma, and alcohol consumption (Mack et al, 2024).

Myths and Misconceptions About OIT

When families first begin exploring oral immunotherapy (OIT), they often experience a mix of hope and hesitation. Some have been told they are not candidates. Others have encountered bold marketing claims. Many feel overwhelmed by the growing number of options.

Dr. Tom Chacko is a board-certified allergist based in Atlanta and founder of Chacko Allergy, where he specializes in personalized care for food allergies, asthma, and immunologic conditions. He is also widely known for his educational social media presence @chacko_allergy, where he shares encouraging patient successes and practical, evidence-based insights to help his audience better understand and manage allergic disease. In our conversation in episode 79 of the *Don't Feed the Fear* podcast (Whitehouse & Chacko, 2026), Dr. Chacko addressed the following questions and misconceptions he hears most often that keep patients feeling stuck.

"My numbers are too high."
According to Dr. Chacko, there is no IgE level that automatically excludes someone from OIT. Higher levels may influence pacing and targets, but not eligibility. High IgE changes the strategy, not the possibility.

"You have to eat it every day forever."
OIT requires ongoing exposure, but not necessarily large daily doses indefinitely. Dr. Chacko explained that maintenance can often be reduced to smaller, consistent doses several times per week. For younger children, this often becomes routine. For older children and teens, the psychological barrier may be greater than the physical one. With support and consistency, dosing often becomes part of daily life.

"Reactions during OIT mean it isn't safe."
Dr. Chacko noted that mild symptoms, particularly gastrointestinal discomfort, are most common. Severe reactions are less common but possible. There has been one reported death of a child undergoing milk OIT. This loss is deeply tragic, exceedingly rare, and highlights a central principle of OIT safety: early recognition of symptoms and prompt, correct use of epinephrine are critical. Published reports indicate that in that case, unfortunately, epinephrine administration was delayed and then not effectively delivered once given (Mondello, 2021).

"We can't do OIT because of EoE."
Eosinophilic esophagitis (EoE) requires careful consideration but is not always an absolute barrier. Dr. Chacko said that he evaluates this individually and if EoE is stable and the allergy significantly impacts quality of life, OIT may still be considered, often with slower progression and lower targets. If EoE symptoms develop, stopping OIT typically allows a return to baseline, but adjustments are often sufficient.

"FDA-approved options are better."
FDA approval reflects regulatory pathways, not necessarily superiority. Dr. Chacko highlighted that food-based OIT does not receive the same funding as pharmaceutical therapies, and the FDA approval process is for medications, not food-based medical regiments. The goal is to align treatments with individual goals, values, and practical realities.

"If my child tolerates baked milk or egg, we don't need OIT."
Tolerance of baked milk or egg does not always translate to tolerance of less heated forms. As Dr. Chacko explained, for those seeking broader dietary freedom, OIT may still be appropriate depending on the patient's trajectory.

"Avoidance is wrong."
Avoidance remains a valid choice. OIT is an option, not an obligation. For some patients, particularly those managing well, avoidance may be appropriate. For younger children, earlier intervention may offer more opportunity to influence long-term immune development. Ultimately, decisions include quality of life and personal values alongside medical details.

"I'm too old/It's too late"

Another common concern among older children and adults is the belief that it may be "too late" to benefit from immunotherapy. Dr. Chacko emphasized that most patients of any age who are motivated and able to follow the treatment consistently can achieve increased tolerance. At the same time, he noted that starting earlier may offer unique advantages. Dr. Chacko said that the only time he encourages patients to take action sooner than later is with very young children. They are more likely to experience more lasting changes at the level of the immune system, with the potential to move beyond tolerance and incorporate the allergen more fully into their diet over time (Vickery et al., 2017). In contrast, older patients typically remain allergic but can still gain meaningful protection through increased tolerance (Whitehouse & Chacko, 2026).

Research on early immunotherapy suggests that there may be meaningful benefits to transitioning children into treatment soon after a failed food introduction. In a real-world study of preschool-aged children undergoing peanut oral immunotherapy, treatment in this younger age group was safe, effective, and unlikely to elicit severe symptoms or reactions. In particular, children who show signs of an allergy following initial early introduction of a food may benefit from prompt treatment, rather than moving into long-term avoidance. Early treatment may help prevent the allergy from becoming more entrenched over time and can take advantage of a developmental window in which the immune system may be more responsive to change (Soller et al., 2019).

"It's what's best for my child."

Dr. Chacko described concerns with parents driven more by parental anxiety than the teen's goals, especially just before the time comes to leave for college. If the patient is not committed, OIT may not be the right fit. Conversely, some children strongly desire relief while parents hesitate. Supporting the child's voice is essential (Whitehouse & Chacko, 2026).

Across conversations with Dr. Chacko and Dr. Jones, a consistent message emerged: know your options, understand your goals, individualize the plan, and be cautious of absolutes. OIT is neither a miracle cure nor a reckless gamble. It is a structured, evidence-informed tool that, when aligned with the right patient and goals, can meaningfully change both immune response and daily life.

Mindset, Meaning, and the Emotional Work of OIT

Before considering OIT, every patient and family needs to consider not only whether they *can*, but whether they *should*. Knowing that younger children may have the best treatment outcomes, parents often feel that they are falling behind, and older kids and adults may feel that they're too late. People naturally translate nuance into self-blame, and UK allergist Professor Adam Fox makes space for that, rather than dismissing it. Prof. Fox spoke gently about the guilt that surfaces when parents of an older child wonder if they waited too long in episode 81 of the *Don't Feed the Fear* podcast (Whitehouse & Fox, 2026). Prof. Fox is pediatric allergist known for multiple roles in allergy leadership, clinical care, and research. He helped lead the way to immunotherapy access for UK patients, and in 2025 Prof. Fox was honored for his contributions to the world of allergy with an OBE (Officer of the Most Excellent Order of the British Empire), a prestigious UK honor awarded by the King.

Prof. Fox acknowledged the very real physical manifestation of stress that can show up as "noise in the system." He noted that biological systems are never still and shifts in eczema, asthma, and the immune system are to be expected. During OIT, mild symptoms often reflect engagement of the immune system, not necessarily danger (Whitehouse & Fox, 2026).

This perspective is supported by research about the impact of teaching patients about OIT "symptoms as positive signals" (SAPS). The approach reframes mild reactions, like an itchy mouth or stomach discomfort, as signs that the immune system is actively engaging and adapting due to treatment. In their study, patients who were taught this framework instead of being taught that their symptoms were "side effects" were less anxious, less likely to contact medical staff for reassurance, less likely to skip or reduce doses, experienced fewer mild symptoms, and showed greater increases in the biological markers associated with successful allergy desensitization. In other words, the story told about symptoms changed not only how patients felt, but how treatment unfolded (Howe et al., 2019).

This refers to minor symptoms, of course. Severe reactions can occur, and OIT patients are carefully trained to recognize and treat them. Prof. Fox reported that many reactions are linked to identifiable cofactors like illness, fatigue, or exercise too soon after dosing (Whitehouse & Fox, 2026). When reactions occur in a controlled setting, families often discover something unexpected: anaphylaxis, while serious, is often more manageable than the catastrophic image they had imagined. That experience can build competence rather than fear.

Prof. Fox has also observed increases in reactions during periods of heightened community stress, such as major sporting events. The neuroimmune connection is not theoretical. When a patient approaches a dose already feelings anxious, the body is more likely to interpret sensations as threat. Some teens even report symptoms before the food touches their tongue. The immune system and nervous system are in constant dialogue. This is why attention to motivation and mindset are crucial. Beginning OIT stressed, afraid, or lacking motivation can make the road tougher than necessary (Whitehouse & Fox, 2026).

Our Mindset Starting Out

When I was first considering OIT for my son, I knew from what I'd read that it was done in a safe and controlled manner, but the thought of feeding him a peanut was hard to wrap my mind around. I had spent years doing the exact opposite, so carefully avoiding and eliminating all risk. And yet, he had also lived through enough reactions to know what that reality looked like.

The question became less about whether a reaction was possible, and more about *when* and *under what conditions*. There was something about the structure of treatment and the data supporting it that helped me feel able to tackle something so daunting. If he was going to react, this was a setting designed to support him through it. (It helped that our OIT doctor's office was attached to a hospital.) If it worked, it could mean fewer reactions over time, less fear, and more safety in daily life.

I worked hard to tame my anxiety and trust the doctor, even though I noticed early in treatment that on most updose days my son's ears would turn red and swell slightly. This subtle change echoed how his ears had looked during past allergic reactions, including ones that were more concerning. Each time it happened during OIT, his doctor examined him closely.

His lungs were clear. His vital signs were stable. We were consistently reassured that this response was not concerning. My son sometimes noticed, but never expressed discomfort with these signs. As a parent with lived experience of severe reactions, I still noticed every little thing. These were visible reminders of past emergencies layered onto a new and unfamiliar process.

As the pattern became more familiar, we needed a way to talk about what was happening that did not automatically pull us into fear. At some point, I began saying that his body was "noticing" the dose. That phrase created space between responding and reacting. It helped differentiate between an effect of treatment and danger.

Framing it this way did not make us careless. We still watched closely and carefully documented everything, but this mindset shifted the emotional tone. These moments became something to observe rather than something to brace against. Slowly, we began to see these signs as hope that his immune system was recognizing the allergen without escalating into an emergency.

As we progressed through treatment, we saw how his body responded and how that response evolved over time. I'll share more of those details as we move through the different stages of the process later in the book.

Explaining OIT to Children

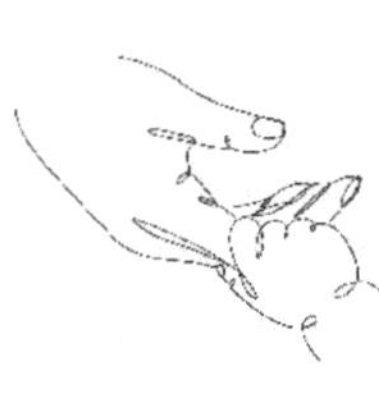

Oral Immunotherapy (OIT) is a treatment where doctors help patients eat tiny, carefully measured amounts of the foods they are allergic to so their bodies can slowly learn to tolerate them. It can feel unusual or a little scary at first, but like learning any new skill, the process happens in small steps. It is important to ensure that children understand that participating in OIT is done safely and carefully under allergist supervision to avoid reactions and epinephrine use.

Below are developmentally attuned ways to explain OIT to children at different ages:

Under 5: Concrete, Simple, and Reassuring
At this age, children think in literal and sensory ways. Keep explanations short and grounded in what they will experience, and specific examples of the benefits of treatment.

You might say:
"The doctor is going to help your body learn that your allergen is safe so it won't have a big allergic reaction. We swallow a small dose at the doctor's office, wait together to make sure it's working, then go home. We do the same thing at home, and rest afterward to teach your body to stay calm. That will help you to eat more foods safely."

Helpful strategies:

- Use familiar, gentle words like "swallow."

- Be honest about how it might feel, and offer comfort: "It might feel funny, but I'll be right there with you."

- Focus on togetherness and routine: "We do the bite, read or play together while we wait, then you get a sticker."

- Acting out the routine with toys can help reduce anxiety. Pretend to eat toy foods. Act out using a syringe to draw up and swallow liquids at home if that is what your doctor will be using to measure and administer the dose. Children often mistake these for needles.

At this age, predictability and adult presence regulate the nervous system more than explanations do.

Ages 5–8: Building Understanding and Mastery

Early elementary children can grasp basic cause-and-effect and often want to know *why*.

You might say:
"Your body thinks certain foods are dangerous, and the OIT will help your immune system practice staying calm. Each dose is like a little step on a journey. Each time you dose it helps your body practice and learn that it doesn't need to have a big allergic reaction."

Helpful additions:

- Compare the process to sports practice or learning to ride a bike. Small steps build skill.

- Let them track progress on a chart or calendar.

- Normalize mixed feelings: "It's okay to feel nervous and excited at the same time."

- Emphasize their role: "You're helping your body learn."

Ages 9–12: More Detail and Collaborative Framing

Older children can handle nuanced explanations and may want specifics about safety and outcomes.

You might say:
"OIT is a special kind of treatment that teaches your immune system to handle foods that you have had allergic reactions to in the past. You start with very small amounts that aren't enough to make you sick, and slowly build up. After each dose, we wait so the doctor can make sure it's working. It's like climbing a hill. You go slowly and carefully, but each step takes you closer to the top."

Helpful approaches:

- Explain the schedule honestly (daily doses at home, regular clinic visits).

- Talk about the importance of monitoring and safety.

- Acknowledge inconvenience or worry and validate feelings.

- Invite them to ask questions and be part of planning: "What would you like to ask the doctor? What might help you feel safe at home during doses?"

Teens: Transparency, Autonomy, and Big-Picture Perspective

Adolescents benefit from direct, respectful conversation, understanding long-term goals, and being part of decisions.

You might say:
"OIT is a treatment that gradually trains your body to tolerate foods that you have had allergic reactions to. It takes time and commitment, and there are some risks, but most reactions are mild. Think of it like training for a big race. Each dose slowly helps your body learn not to react, which will make you safer and protect you against allergic reactions."

Helpful strategies:

- Encourage real dialogue about risks, benefits, and lifestyle considerations.

- Discuss the teen's goals: "What foods would you like to be able to eat safely?" "Are there things you'd like to do or accomplish that food allergies have made more difficult?"

- Include them in planning and routines at home to build ownership and confidence.

The Tolerance Induction Program

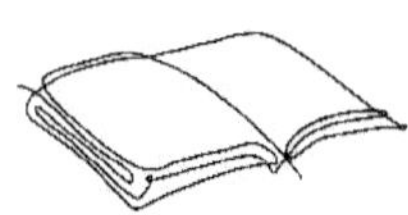

The Tolerance Induction Program (TIP) developed by Dr. Inderpal Randhawa is another widely recognized approach to food allergy treatment. While it shares the core principle of gradual exposure to allergens, the broader context surrounding TIP is somewhat different from other models.

Dr. Randhawa has published aspects of this work, but his program is privately operated through the Food Allergy Institute's locations across California. It has largely developed outside of the standard academic and collaborative frameworks that guide much of allergy research and clinical practice. As a result, less peer-reviewed data and fewer publicly available outcomes exist compared to treatments like OIT. This does not diminish the experiences of patients who have participated in TIP, many of whom report meaningful improvements, but it does mean that families may encounter more variability in the type, sources, and amount of information available when considering this option. The goal throughout this book is to offer a clear understanding of the landscape so families can make their own informed decisions.

What is TIP?

When asked to explain the origin of TIP in episode 90 of the *Don't Feed the Fear* podcast, Dr. Randhawa noted that his professional experience with research and development in medicine motivated him to consider food allergy treatment through the analysis of large volumes of immune data and identify highly individualized immune profiles. That systems-level, data-driven mindset shaped how he created TIP (Whitehouse & Randhawa, 2026).

According to his description, TIP begins with extensive immune profiling. He reports running hundreds of biomarkers per patient, including blood tests, skin testing, patch testing, and lung-based assessments, in order to build a detailed immune "baseline landscape." That data is fed into proprietary machine learning systems that generate a risk profile for each patient. Families are told which foods are predicted to trigger anaphylaxis, the relative severity of those reactions, and which foods may be tolerated.

From there, the core of TIP utilizes "biosimilar proteins." Rather than starting by dosing the primary allergen directly, the program introduces proteins that are structurally similar to the allergen but are not the primary trigger. The aim, as Dr. Randhawa described it, is to lower the immune system's reactivity to the main allergen before that allergen is ever consumed. He reports that patients often begin by consuming these biosimilar proteins for a period of time, and once immune markers have shifted they transition to direct introduction of the primary allergen. For example, someone allergic to peanuts may start dosing with other legumes which contains proteins of a similar structure.

For those with multiple allergens, TIP is described as downregulating all of these simultaneously, with the goal of remission with full dietary inclusion. Dr. Randhawa describes patients ultimately consuming large, age-appropriate servings of previously reactive foods without restriction (Whitehouse & Randhawa, 2026).

Dr. Randhawa reported a 99% success rate and a 1% adverse side effects rate. He also states that the program does not exclude patients based on severity or comorbid conditions, including high IgE levels, severe eczema, asthma, eosinophilic esophagitis (EoE), or mast cell disorders (Whitehouse & Randhawa, 2026). Published data from Dr. Randhawa and colleagues describe evidence of sustained unresponsiveness in patients undergoing milk immunotherapy through TIP, as well as detailed clinical characterization of nut allergy populations treated within this model (Randhawa & Marsteller, 2024; Marsteller et al., 2021). "Sustained unresponsiveness" in this context means they demonstrated that the immune system can handle large, infrequent doses of an allergen without an allergic reaction, even after stopping daily consumption for a period (e.g., 4 weeks or more).

Is TIP different from OIT?

Critics of TIP have challenged claims made about the limitations and risks of OIT, stating that certain characterizations are not consistent with their clinical experience or confirmed by publicly available data. Others have raised concerns about transparency, noting that TIP protocols are not publicly available in the way academic research protocols typically are. Cost has also been a point of discussion, as the program can represent a significant financial investment for families, typically beyond the costs of OIT.

Dr. Randhawa framed these dynamics differently. He described his work as intentionally built outside of what he calls the "medical industrial complex," meaning it was not developed through traditional pharmaceutical funding channels, venture capital, or university-based trials. In his view, that independence allowed for faster innovation but also required him to build research, data systems, and infrastructure internally. He pointed to safety data and regulatory oversight through informed consent processes and institutional review structures as evidence of accountability (Whitehouse & Randhawa, 2026).

These differing perspectives are part of the broader landscape, and it is important to be aware that TIP generates strong opinions across the food allergy community.

Common Questions

Many families considering TIP want to know specifically in comparison to OIT how this approach differs, what the short- and long-term safety outcomes are, what remission means biologically, and how durable it is over time.

These are appropriate questions, and the things we want to know about any treatment that requires time, financial, and emotional investment. Since TIP does not engage with the larger allergy treatment community or share its data in the same format, it can be more difficult to find clear answers to some of these questions.

The Mental Health Landscape of TIP

Families who pursue TIP often describe achieving food tolerance or "remission," as well as something else that is harder to quantify: a rapid shift in perceived control. Dr. Randhawa spoke about how anxiety levels in families appear to decrease once they feel they understand their child's risk profile and have immediate clinical access to support. Whether that psychological shift comes from the biological changes, the data transparency, the intensity of follow-up, or the experience of "wins" along the way is difficult to separate. What is clear is that psychological factors are deeply intertwined with medical decisions and experiences.

Even if the medical architecture of TIP differs from oral immunotherapy, the lived experience of it will feel familiar to many families. Dr. Randhawa shared clearly that the biological strategy behind TIP is not the same as OIT. The sequencing of proteins is different, the immune modeling is different, and the stated goal is remission rather than maintenance. Those distinctions matter medically (Whitehouse & Randhawa, 2026).

Behaviorally, the daily reality for a child and parent often looks similar. The routines, travel, scheduled doses, monitoring, follow up appointments, financial commitment, time off work, rearranged school schedules, and impact on siblings are similar. Emotionally, the fear and anxiety about consuming allergens, possible side effects and reactions, and motivation required to see the program through also remain. As with every other treatment option discussed in this workbook, there are individuals who describe TIP as life-changing, others who did not complete it or did not experience the hoped-for outcome, and still others who experienced twists and turns along the way but felt that their individual gains were worthwhile.

Controversy can be uncomfortable and can also be an exciting sign that a field is evolving and growing. Your task is not to solve that controversy. It is to decide what aligns with your values, your resources, your risk tolerance, and your goals.

Sarah's Experience with the Tolerance Induction Program (TIP)

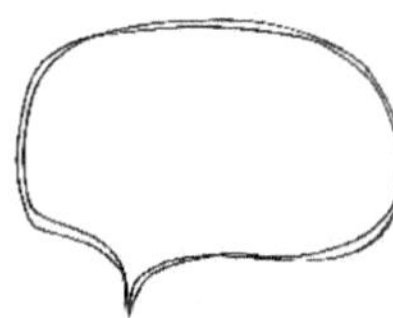

Sarah Danna is a young adult who shares her life with food allergies and mast cell activation syndrome (MCAS) as @sarahandspices. She shared her experience with TIP in episode 91 of the *Don't Feed the Fear* podcast (Whitehouse & Danna, 2026).

Finding Her Way to Treatment

Diagnosed as a toddler, Sarah grew up navigating food allergies as part of daily life. But in her early teens, her symptoms became more complex, with frequent reactions not only to food, but also to environmental triggers and even clothing. At one point, her safe foods narrowed to just thirteen, and her world felt increasingly restricted. With medical support and efforts to stabilize her system, her symptoms eventually improved.

She discovered the Tolerance Induction Program (TIP) through social media and, after a consultation, decided to move forward. Looking back, Sarah said that her decision felt less about choosing between options and more about deciding whether to try treatment at all. At the time she made the decision, she knew little about other immunotherapy options.

The Treatment Experience

A consistent theme in Sarah's journey is taking things one step at a time. This mindset, shaped by her upbringing, allowed her to focus on the next step rather than the full scope of treatment. TIP involved both clinic-based care and structured routines at home. Clinic visits often included food challenges, monitoring, and dose adjustments, while her daily routine incorporated sublingual immunotherapy (SLIT), regular intake of maintenance foods, and carefully timed micro-doses. What initially felt overwhelming became manageable as she developed routines and systems to support the process.

One of her most meaningful milestones was passing a peanut challenge after a history of anaphylaxis to them. While peanuts were not a preferred food, the relief from constant fear of cross-contact brought a significant shift in her daily life. Each milestone, even small ones, expanded what felt possible.

Adapting Along the Way

About two years into treatment, Sarah's path shifted when her care team recognized that some treatment reactions did not align with expected patterns. Further evaluation led to her MCAS diagnosis, helping explain why certain foods remained difficult to treat. She ultimately reached tolerance to nine foods through TIP, and will continue to work with them to address remaining symptoms and allergens with a plan adapted in response to her MCAS diagnosis and symptoms. Her experience reflects the reality that treatment is not always linear and often requires adjustment.

Perspective and Moving Forward

When Sarah speaks to others considering treatment, she emphasizes that there is no single "right" path. Sarah's story reflects both the progress and complexity of food allergy treatment, and the possibility of building a full, meaningful life alongside it.

Natalie's Experience: Complexity, Courage, and Choosing Treatment

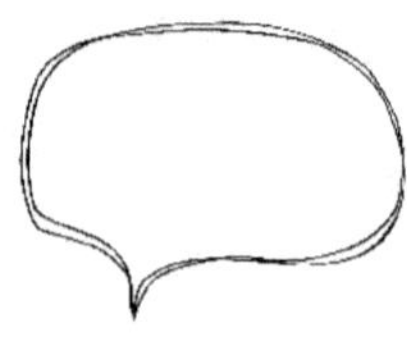

Natalie Grijalva is the voice behind the Instagram account @createlikeamom, which she originally started to share creativity as a form of expression in motherhood, and ended up shifting to food allergy and Kawasaki disease content as her parenting journey unfolded. She shared her family's experience with food allergies, Kawasaki disease, and TIP in episode 92 of the *Don't Feed the Fear* podcast (Whitehouse and Grijalva, 2026).

The youngest of Natalie's three children, the only one with food allergies, brought with him a level of medical complexity that shifted everything for the family. From early on, Natalie had the sense that something wasn't quite right with his health. By eight months old, after a frightening reaction to formula that sent them rushing to urgent care, she knew she was entering a season of parenting that required vigilance, advocacy, and a steep learning curve.

Getting a dairy allergy diagnosis wasn't straightforward, nor was building a trustworthy medical support team or social community due frequent military relocation. Much of what she learned came from experience and other parents. During one of those moves, her son suffered a severe anaphylactic reaction. Seeing her son go limp and administering epinephrine in a hotel hallway became one of the defining experiences of her early years as an allergy parent. It was terrifying, and like so many families, it left a lasting imprint.

As her son got older, it became clear that this wasn't something he would simply outgrow. His allergy levels continued to rise, and daily life felt increasingly restrictive. Food involved ongoing risk management. Travel was complicated. Social experiences were limited. The weight of constant vigilance was exhausting.

Considering a Different Path

Natalie began researching treatment options, including both OIT and TIP. She watched, listened, followed other families sharing their experiences, and weighed the realities carefully. She prepared herself for a significant investment of time, finances, and daily care and attention to the dosing routine.

Natalie was living in California when she added her son to the TIP waitlist, wanting to take advantage of their close proximity to the program. Just as he reached the top of the list, the family found out that the military was relocating them to the east coast. Natalie held off treatment until they were settled, accepted that the family would have to take on considerable financial debt in order to fund TIP, and committed to the trips back to California every 3 months. Their first appointment was an extensive intake including detailed history, comprehensive testing, and careful consideration of how her child had actually responded to foods in real life. Then, during the second visit that's known as "launch week," treatment began.

Natalie appreciated the thorough, gradual, and methodical approach at TIP. She explained that treatment begins far from the allergen itself, in her son's case with amino acid formula, and progresses over time toward more recognizable forms of the food. For Natalie's son, this meant moving through a wide range of exposures: specialized formulas, then milks and yogurts from different animals (camel, donkey, sheep), then increasingly recognizable dairy products. Challenges along the way included taste aversions, mild symptoms like throat itching, the day-to-day work of dosing, monitoring, and of course the frequent and expensive travel (Whitehouse and Grijalva, 2026).

Treatment in the Context of Real Life

About halfway through their journey, life interrupted in a profound way. Natalie's son became critically ill and was eventually diagnosed with Kawasaki disease, a rare and serious condition that affects the blood vessels and can impact the heart. What followed were a prolonged hospitalization, significant uncertainty, slow recovery, and ongoing cardiac complications that continue to require monitoring. Research has also found that children with common allergic diseases may have an increased risk of developing Kawasaki disease, underscoring the complex and not yet fully understood relationships within the immune system (Wei et al., 2014).

Treatment for food allergies paused, then with careful planning and attention from TIP, resumed without issue. One of the most meaningful aspects of Natalie's experience was the flexibility within the treatment process. This allowed her son to start back on treatment at a smaller and safe dose following his health issues, and gradually return to progression when it was safe to do so.

Where They Are Now

Nearly three years into treatment and 8 years old, Natalie's son is tolerating boiled cow milk. His medical issues added to the overall time it will take him to move through the TIP program, and there are still unknowns related to his long-term cardiac health. The journey has required immense sacrifice, including financial strain, time, and emotional energy. Natalie feels strongly that it has all been worth it for the added safety and possibility that TIP has brought.

What Natalie Wants Other Families to Know

Natalie is careful not to present her path as the *only* path. She is thoughtful about encouraging other families to do their own research, explore multiple options, connect with other families in treatment, and consider what aligns best with their individual circumstances. She is also adamant that if a patient is having trouble avoiding allergens and preventing reactions, these options are worth the investment (Whitehouse and Grijalva, 2026).

Explaining TIP to Children

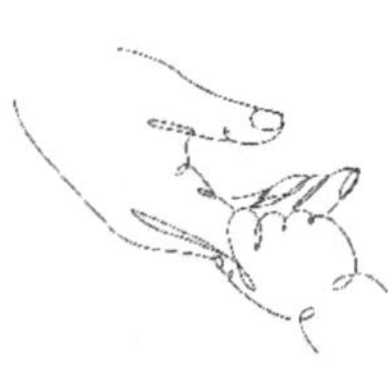 The Tolerance Induction Program (TIP) is a treatment designed to help children build tolerance to foods they are allergic to, using carefully measured doses under medical supervision. Children are supported both in the clinic and at home to safely eat foods that once caused allergic reactions. Children should understand, at an age-appropriate level, that daily dosing, appointments, and travel will be part of the experience.

Under 5: Concrete, Simple, and Reassuring

At this age, children think in literal and sensory ways. Keep explanations short and specific.

You might say:
"The doctor is going to teach your body not to react to your allergens anymore by showing it that these foods are safe. We swallow the medicine, wait together to make sure it's working, then go home."

Helpful strategies:

- Use simple, reassuring words like "swallow" instead of "doses" or "therapy."

- Emphasize togetherness: "I'll be right there with you."

- Prepare them through play therapy with toys or pretend foods.

- Predictable routines help them feel safe: "We go, we taste a little, wait, then get a sticker."

- Incorporate play with oral syringes if they will be used for dosing. Many children mistake these as needles, so if they will be used it is helpful to clarify in advance.

Ages 5–8: Building Understanding and Mastery

Early elementary children can understand cause-and-effect and like to know why.

You might say:
"Your body thinks certain foods are dangerous, but TIP helps your body practice staying calm. Each taste is like a little step on a journey, and over time your body learns it doesn't need to have a reaction to protect you."

Helpful additions:
- Compare it to practicing a skill like riding a bike or learning a new game.

- Track progress with a chart, stickers, or calendar.

- Normalize nervousness and excitement: "It's okay to feel both at the same time."

- Reinforce empowerment: "You are helping your body learn."

Ages 9–12: More Detail and Collaborative Framing

Older children can handle nuanced explanations and want details about how and why.

You might say:
"TIP is a program that teaches your body to tolerate your allergens. You start by swallowing very small amounts and gradually increase them to teach your body not to react. It's like climbing a hill. Each step takes you closer to the top, and you go at a pace your body can handle."

Helpful approaches:

- Explain daily routines at home and clinic visits honestly.

- Discuss safety procedures and why monitoring is important.

- Invite questions and input on routines at home: "What makes it easier for you to take your tiny tastes?"

- Acknowledge challenges while emphasizing progress.

Teens: Transparency, Autonomy, and Big-Picture Perspective

Adolescents need direct, respectful conversation and want to understand long-term goals.

You might say:
"TIP helps your body slowly learn to eat your allergens without reacting. It takes time, effort, and commitment, and will make you safer. Think of it like training for a big adventure. You're taking it step by step, learning how your body responds, and gaining more freedom over time."

Helpful strategies:

- Encourage discussion of risks, benefits, and lifestyle impact.

- Be honest about the chance of symptoms, usually mild, if they ask.

- Ask about their personal goals: "Which foods would you like to eat safely?"

- Include them in planning doses, snacks, and routines to build ownership and confidence.

- Emphasize that setbacks are normal and part of learning.

Sublingual Immunotherapy (SLIT)

 Like other forms of immunotherapy, the goal of sublingual immunotherapy (SLIT) is to gradually retrain the immune system over time. Small amounts of either environmental or food allergens are placed under the tongue and absorbed through the oral mucosa before being swallowed or spit out, depending on the protocol recommended by the provider. It is typically done at home, tends to involve fewer immediate demands around appointments, and is often perceived and experienced as a gentler entry point into the world of immunotherapy.

For those weighing not only the medical aspects of treatment but also the emotional, logistical, and developmental fit, SLIT can represent a meaningful alternative. It does not remove the need for consistency, patience, or thoughtful decision-making, but it may shift how those demands are experienced in daily life.

For environmental allergies, SLIT has been used for many years and is well-established as a treatment option. In the context of food allergies, it is considered a more gradual and often more conservative approach compared to oral immunotherapy (OIT). While SLIT may be a slower path to desensitization, it is often valued for its safety profile, flexibility, and effectiveness (Ilyasova & Kim, 2026).

How It Works

In episode 89 of the *Don't Feed the Fear* podcast, Dr. Nikhila Schroeder pointed out that describing SLIT as "allergy drops under the tongue" is incomplete (Whitehouse & Schroeder, 2026). Dr. Schroeder is double board certified in allergy & immunology and pediatrics, and is the founder of Allergenuity Health, where she provides personalized, integrative care for individuals and families navigating allergic conditions. She is known for her innovative approach focusing on SLIT in food allergy care.

Dr. Schroeder explained that SLIT utilizes the oral mucosa, the immune-rich surface inside the mouth. When tiny amounts of allergen protein are placed there, specialized immune cells called "dendritic cells" sample that protein and carry the information back to the lymph nodes. Dr. Schroeder beautifully summarizes the simple message they deliver: *Look again. This is food, not a virus or bacterium. This is not a threat.*

Dr. Schroeder described this as going back to basics. Babies explore the world through their mouths. They put fingers, toys, clothing, and everything else they can reach into that space. The oral mucosa is designed to promote tolerance. It is one of the most naturally tolerant and most immunologically sophisticated surfaces in the body. SLIT harnesses that biology by presenting the immune system with the very protein it has misclassified and inviting it to reconsider, taking advantage of a natural pathway for immune education (Whitehouse & Schroeder, 2026).

Who Can Use SLIT?

One of the most important points Dr. Schroeder made is that almost anyone with a food or environmental allergy can be considered for SLIT. Almost all patients can benefit from it regardless of age, IgE levels, sensitivity, past reaction history, or other allergic conditions (asthma, eczema, and eosinophilic esophagitis). For babies who cannot "hold" drops under their tongues, there are creative approaches. Drops can be placed along the gums or in the vestibular area inside the cheek. Dosing volumes are small and viscous, so much of the protein still interacts with the oral mucosa before being swallowed. The flexibility of SLIT is one of its defining strengths. Because it is delivered in liquid form, the dose can always be lowered. If a child develops oral itching or an eczema flare, the liquid can be further diluted and the protocol can be slowed.

Safety and Symptoms

In research and in long-standing clinical practices, anaphylaxis from SLIT dosing is exceedingly rare. Oral itching is the most common symptom. Occasionally, there may be mild eczema flares. These usually resolve with slower escalation or small adjustments in dosing. SLIT is generally considered to have a strong safety profile with meaningful efficacy (Ilyasova & Kim, 2026).

In Dr. Schroeder's training and decade of practice, she has never seen anaphylaxis from SLIT dosing. That does not mean vigilance disappears. It means the risk profile is fundamentally different from higher dose oral immunotherapy (Whitehouse & Schroeder, 2026).

Dr. Allison Freeman echoed this distinction in episode 85 of the *Don't Feed the Fear* podcast (Whitehouse & Freeman, 2026). Dr. Freeman is a board certified allergist and immunologist practicing in Virginia and specializing in immunotherapy and innovative treatment approaches for both environmental and food allergies. She is known for her practical, personalized approach to care and her openness to the psychological and emotional impact of living with food allergies and undergoing treatment.

Dr. Freeman said that while SLIT can be a powerful standalone treatment, she also utilizes it as a bridge to oral immunotherapy (OIT). Some patients and families have difficulty with the side effects and safety precautions required by OIT including a no exercise window (usually 2 hours), and strict food timing rules for dosing. Some SLIT providers require shorter post-dose precautions, and it typically has fewer and more mild symptoms, creating a lower lifestyle burden that can make it more accessible.

That difference is particularly meaningful for teenagers who struggle with structured treatment. Dr. Freeman reported that she has seen many OIT reactions occur when teens dose late, skip meals, rush out the door, or head to parties. When treatment starts to conflict with a teenager's autonomy and social life, adherence suffers. SLIT fits more naturally into that developmental stage, particularly if immunotherapy is a new addition to the routine (Whitehouse & Freeman, 2026).

What Can SLIT Achieve?

Historically, SLIT has been framed as the "lower goal" immunotherapy option, providing protection from accidental exposures or cross contact, sometimes referred to as "bite safety." Dr. Schroeder emphasized that SLIT can go beyond that. While many families begin with the goal of reducing the risk of anaphylaxis from trace exposures, some patients progress to tolerating much larger amounts of their allergens. Not everyone chooses to incorporate those foods into daily life, but it can be achieved (Whitehouse & Schroeder, 2026).

According to Dr. Freeman, research shows that after one year of food-based SLIT, the majority of children can tolerate around 100 milligrams of their trigger food in a supervised challenge. With additional years, those thresholds increase. Ten to thirty milligrams may cover many "may contain" and shared equipment exposures. One to two bites may become realistic within one to two years of consistent treatment for many children (Whitehouse & Freeman, 2026; Kim & Burks, 2020). For families who have lived in fear of every precautionary label or the risk of cross-contact in everyday settings, that threshold is life-changing.

SLIT can also be combined with other approaches. Some families begin with SLIT and later transition to oral therapy. Others transition to SLIT after difficulty with OIT. Some use a combination of both treatments for different allergens. Dr. Freeman even shared that co-treating multiple nuts simultaneously using food-based protocols such as nut puff snacks can increase convenience, allow broader coverage, and decrease cost and treatment complexity. She uses these instead of liquids to dissolve under the tongue and provide a consistently measured dose.

Extract-based SLIT offers precision and convenience but can be expensive. Food-based SLIT can be more affordable but requires mixing at home. Each model has trade-offs. Creative physicians are working to make more options accessible so that each patient can choose what will work for them (Whitehouse & Freeman, 2026).

Why Is SLIT Overlooked?

In episode 78 of the *Don't Feed the Fear* podcast, Dr. Doug Jones spoke about the attention economy within medicine (Whitehouse & Jones, 2026). Treatments that produce dramatic numbers or visible ingestion often attract more headlines, and researchers developing these treatments anticipated that incorporating allergens into the diet would be the goal for many patients. Dr. Jones' time and experience have shown that safety is often patients' number one priority. He has seen interest in and attention to SLIT increase over time, and he expects that it will be a more accessible option moving forward (Whitehouse & Jones, 2026).

Dr. Freeman notes that many allergists are waiting for larger, placebo-controlled trials before incorporating SLIT into their clinics (Whitehouse & Freeman, 2026). Studies currently underway such as those led by Dr. Edwin Kim at Chapel Hill are expected to provide additional clarity about long-term outcomes and protection levels. As that data accumulates, broader adoption may follow.

The Psychological Fit

From a psychological perspective, the emotional layer is often overlooked but contributes significantly to treatment adherence and outcomes. SLIT may be uniquely well-suited for anxious children and families who carry trauma around food. For some, even holding a bottle labeled with the allergen is a major step.

Extract-based SLIT looks and feels like medicine. It does not taste or smell like the allergen, which allows it to serve as a bridge between total avoidance and treatment (Whitehouse & Schroeder, 2026).

Practical Realities

SLIT induction is typically faster than oral therapy. Maintenance can often be reached within four to seven visits. Dosing takes minutes, and travel may be less or even unnecessary after the initial appointment, with more providers offering virtual SLIT updose appointments.

Multiple allergens can be treated simultaneously without multiplying gastrointestinal side effects in the way oral immunotherapy can. Despite SLIT's safety, careful adherence to the routine and allergist's instructions is still important. Precautions around illness and missed doses will still apply, and communication with your allergist is essential.

Cost remains a barrier in some settings, especially for extract-based protocols. Food-based SLIT can reduce that burden but may require more hands-on involvement from families. This will vary widely by practice and allergens being treated (Whitehouse & Freeman, 2026).

A Treatment With Range

For some toddlers, OIT may offer the best chance at full desensitization and even tolerance over time. For some older children, SLIT may be the most sustainable long-term strategy. For many, a combination approach makes sense.

Daily free eating or even a cure are ideal, of course. Yet SLIT offers what many families want the most: a safety buffer and a reduction in catastrophic risk, which gives them the ability to eat and live more freely and calmly. Clinical trials have demonstrated that SLIT can safely increase tolerance to allergens over time, even in young children, making it a reasonable option for families prioritizing safety and consistency over rapid dose escalation (Keet et al., 2012)

SLIT may not be right for everyone, but it is a far more powerful option than its reputation suggests.

Sublingual Immunotherapy (SLIT) for Environmental Allergies

SLIT is widely used to address environmental allergies in addition to food allergies. Allergen extracts or tablets are placed under the tongue where the allergen interacts with immune cells in the oral mucosa. Those cells process the allergen and help recalibrate the immune response over time. The safety profile of SLIT for environmental allergens is strong. Most side effects are localized and mild, such as oral itching or throat irritation, according to Dr. Freeman (Whitehouse & Freeman, 2026). Systemic reactions are rare, which makes SLIT particularly appealing for those who want treatment without the routine of injections or frequent office visits (Castellana & Chiappetta, 2025).

Dr. Freeman also noted that SLIT may be especially helpful for children who are needle averse or for families who live far from their allergist's office. The convenience of home dosing increases accessibility and adherence for many patients.

SLIT for environmental allergies offers convenience but has several limitations. In the U.S., options are limited to a small number of FDA-approved tablets for single allergens (such as for ragweed, certain grasses, and dust mites). Clinicians can mix custom liquid drops with allergen extracts or order them from outside suppliers, but this can be more costly. In addition, insurance coverage often requires prior authorization or declines coverage for SLIT (Whitehouse & Freeman, 2026).

Explaining SLIT to Children

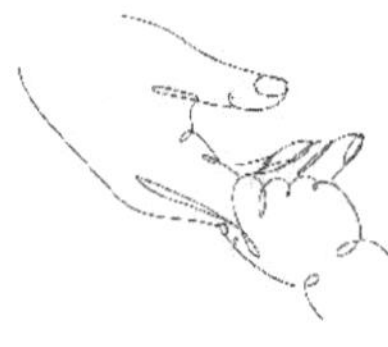 Sublingual Immunotherapy, or SLIT, is a treatment where tiny drops of an allergen are placed under the tongue to help your body get used to foods or environmental triggers over time. SLIT is taken at home every day, and can be swallowed or held under the tongue and spit out.

Under 5: Concrete, Simple, and Reassuring

Young children think literally and focus on immediate experiences.

You might say:
"You put a tiny drop under your tongue every day to teach your body that this isn't dangerous."

Helpful strategies:

- Use simple, concrete language like "tiny drop"

- Keep routines predictable: same time, same place each day.

- Stay close during dosing to provide reassurance.

- Play therapy at home with drops of any liquid can help kids feel more comfortable and practice holding the liquid under the tongue. Find out if your child's drops will be administered with an oral syringe or special vial/bottle, and do your best to mimic this.

Ages 5–8: Building Understanding and Mastery

Children in early elementary school can grasp basic cause-and-effect and enjoy participating actively.

You might say:
"SLIT helps your body practice staying calm when it sees foods or allergens that used to make you sick. Every day, you put a tiny drop under your tongue. Your body is learning not to have a reaction step-by-step, like practicing a sport."

Helpful strategies:

- Let them track doses with a calendar or sticker chart.

- Encourage questions and curiosity about how the treatment works.

- Normalize mixed feelings: excitement and nervousness can coexist.

- Emphasize their role: "You are helping your body learn."

Ages 9–12: More Detail and Collaborative Framing

Older children can understand nuances, schedules, and why monitoring is important.

You might say:
"SLIT is a daily treatment that helps your immune system learn to tolerate allergens. You start with very small doses under your tongue, and over time, your body learns not to react."

Helpful strategies:

- Discuss daily routines and clinic check-ins honestly.

- Explain possible mild reactions and how to manage them.

- Invite input on integrating dosing into school and home routines.

- Emphasize progress over perfection: "Each day is a small step forward."

Teens: Transparency, Autonomy, and Goal-Oriented Framing

Adolescents need direct, respectful conversation about risks, benefits, and goals.

You might say:
"SLIT is done daily to gradually train your body not to react to allergens. You'll put the drops under your tongue and hold them there, and special cells retrain your immune system not to react. Think of it like an athletic training program. By practicing every day, you gain more control and confidence, and over time, your body reacts less."

Helpful strategies:

- Encourage discussion of personal goals: "Which foods or triggers matter most to you?"

- Collaborate on planning dosing, timing, and management of mild symptoms.

- Connect daily routines to the bigger picture: improved freedom and safety.

Subcutaneous Immunotherapy (SCIT) or "Allergy Shots"

 Subcutaneous immunotherapy (SCIT), often referred to as "allergy shots," is one of the most well-known and widely used forms of allergy treatment. While it is not used for food allergies, your doctor may recommend treating environmental allergies before or in conjunction with immunotherapy.

Environmental immunotherapy is fundamentally different from symptom management with maintenance medications. Rather than blocking histamine after the body has reacted, immunotherapy works upstream. It addresses the immune system's misclassification of pollen, dust mites, mold, animal dander, insects, or other allergen as dangerous invaders. Immunotherapy introduces those same allergens in controlled, carefully measured amounts over time so that the immune system can relearn.

Subcutaneous immunotherapy (SCIT) has strong evidence supporting its effectiveness in reducing allergy symptoms and medication use, while also improving quality of life. It is generally considered safe when administered appropriately, though local and occasional systemic reactions can occur (Dhami et al., 2017).

Nothing New

In an episode of the *Don't Feed the Fear* podcast titled, "Immunotherapy Options for Environmental Allergies," Dr. Manisha Relan explained that SCIT is one of the most established treatments in allergy medicine, having been used for over a century (Whitehouse & Relan, 2026). Dr. Relan is a board-certified pediatrician and allergist/immunologist specializing in food allergy prevention and anaphylaxis. In addition to her clinical work, Dr. Relan is known for her educational and advocacy work including her content on social media @pedsallergymd and her role in 101 Before One, an evidence-based baby-led weaning program.

Dr. Relan explained that in SCIT treatment, small but gradually increasing amounts of allergen extract are injected under the skin, typically in the upper arm. These injections are administered in a medical setting because systemic reactions, while uncommon, are possible. The process begins with an individualized build-up phase. Patients usually receive weekly injections, with each dose slightly stronger than the last. This phase can last several months, depending on the protocol and how quickly the patient escalates. Once the target maintenance dose is reached, the schedule shifts to maintenance injections, often every two to four weeks for a duration of three to five years.

Dr. Relan emphasized that SCIT is highly effective for allergic rhinitis, allergic asthma, and venom allergy. Many patients experience substantial reduction in nasal congestion, sneezing, itchy eyes, coughing, wheezing, and eczema. Over time, SCIT can reduce medication reliance and improve overall quality of life. For some, it alters the long-term trajectory of allergic disease, decreasing the likelihood that seasonal allergies will progress to asthma. The trade-off is that SCIT requires regular injections at in-office visits, followed by an observation (typically 30 minutes) to monitor for systemic reactions. For those juggling work, school, and extracurriculars, this time commitment can be significant.

Dr. Relan noted that individuals with uncontrolled asthma, unstable cardiac status, or unstable blood pressure may not be good candidates for SCIT due to the risk of having a severe allergic reaction. There is also the emotional component to consider. Weekly injections can be stressful, painful, and scary. Even when the shots are well-tolerated, the involvement of needles can carry anticipatory anxiety. Still, for many practitioners and patients, SCIT is a trusted treatment option because of its long track record and strong evidence base (Whitehouse & Relan, 2026).

Explaining SCIT (Allergy Shots) to Children at Different Ages

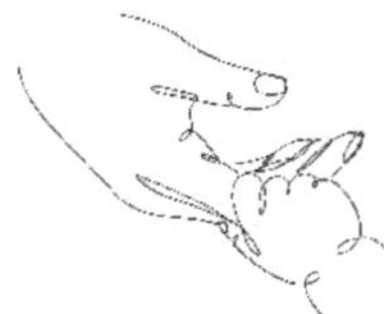

Subcutaneous Immunotherapy (SCIT), often called "allergy shots," can feel intimidating, especially because it involves injections and regular clinic visits with wait time after administration. If you feel anxious about the injections, that's human, but remember that your tension can impact your child.

Below are developmentally attuned ways to explain SCIT to children at different ages.

Under 5: Concrete, Simple, and Reassuring

SCIT isn't usually recommended for kids this young. At this age, children think in very literal and sensory ways. Keep explanations short and grounded in what they will experience.

You might say:

"The doctor is going to give your body tiny bits of the things that make your nose itchy and sneezy. It helps your body learn that those things aren't dangerous. It's a quick poke in your arm, and then we wait together to make sure your body feels okay before we go home."

Helpful strategies:

- Use simple words like "quick poke" rather than "injection."
- Be honest that it may sting briefly and give a plan for managing discomfort.
- Emphasize togetherness: "I'll be right there with you."
- Focus on routine: "We go, we do the poke, we wait, then we go home."
- Play therapy by acting this out at home in advance with toys may help kids prepare.

At this age, predictability regulates the nervous system more than information does.

Ages 6–8: Building Understanding and Mastery

Children in early elementary school can understand basic cause and effect. They often want to know *why*.

You might say:

"Your immune system is a really good protector, but it's getting confused about things like pollen (or dust, pets, etc.). The allergy shots give your body very tiny amounts of that thing so it can get used to it and practice staying calm. Over time, your body learns it doesn't need to react so big."

Helpful additions:

- Compare it to practice in sports or learning to read. Repetition builds skill.
- Let them help track progress on a calendar or sticker chart.
- Invite questions and answer them simply but honestly.
- Normalize mixed feelings: "It's okay to feel nervous about shots and excited about getting better."

This age benefits from empowerment: *"You're helping train your body."*

Ages 9–12: More Detail and Collaborative Framing

Older children can handle more nuanced explanations and may want specifics about safety and effectiveness.

You might say:

"Allergy shots are a type of treatment called immunotherapy. Instead of just treating symptoms, they try to change how your immune system responds. You'll start with very small doses and slowly build up. After each shot, we stay at the doctor's office so they can make sure your body handles it well."

Helpful approaches:

- Discuss the anticipated schedule honestly (weekly build-up, then maintenance).
- Explain why waiting 30 minutes after the shot is important and plan how to spend the time.
- Acknowledge inconvenience and discomfort, and validate frustration.
- Invite them into shared decision-making where appropriate.

At this stage, respecting autonomy strengthens trust.

Teens: Transparency and Autonomy

Adolescents need direct, respectful conversation. They are capable of understanding risks, benefits, and long-term goals.

You might say:

"SCIT requires consistency and time, but for many people it can significantly reduce symptoms and medication needs. Risks are very low, and it is done in a medical setting to monitor for safety after each injection."

Invite real dialogue:

- "What concerns you most?"
- "How does this fit with your schedule?"
- "What would make this feel manageable?"

Teens benefit from collaborative planning and shared values rather than fear or directive reassurance.

SCIT or SLIT for Environmental Allergies

Both SCIT and SLIT aim to retrain the immune system. Both can reduce symptom severity, improve asthma control, and decrease reliance on medications. Both require consistency over years rather than weeks. The differences lie in route, logistics, and lifestyle fit.

In episode 73 of the *Don't Feed the Fear* podcast, Dr. Manisha Relan clarified that SCIT has the longest track record and most robust data supporting its efficacy. It requires ongoing in-office injections and observation periods. SLIT offers a needle-free, home-based alternative with an excellent safety profile and greater day to day flexibility, but slower progress and potentially less durable outcomes. It is also not as widely available as SCIT (Whitehouse & Relan, 2026).

Dr. Relan emphasized that patients who choose to do SLIT for environmental allergies may not already have an epinephrine device available, but should acquire one when beginning treatment. This is because dosing is done daily at home, as opposed to SCIT, which is always done in the office with careful monitoring.

Many patients notice improvement within the first year including milder nasal and eye symptoms and fewer asthma exacerbations. Spring may feel less overwhelming. But Dr. Relan described the bigger picture that she wants patients to understand. SCIT and SLIT can create a shift from daily symptom control to a long-term change. The results of that shift can ripple outward into better sleep, fewer missed work/school days, reduced anxiety about outdoor activities, and less constant vigilance during peak seasons (Whitehouse & Relan, 2026). Considering immunotherapy for environmental allergens can be a quality of life decision.

As with all treatment decisions, the choice should depend on individual factors including age, severity of symptoms, coexisting asthma, family schedule, geographic access to care, financial factors, and patient preference. As you know by now, no form of immunotherapy is a quick fix. Whether using SCIT or SLIT, treatment typically continues for three to five years to achieve lasting immune modification. The goal is durable change, not just seasonal relief.

SLIT for Environmental Allergies: The Part We Almost Missed

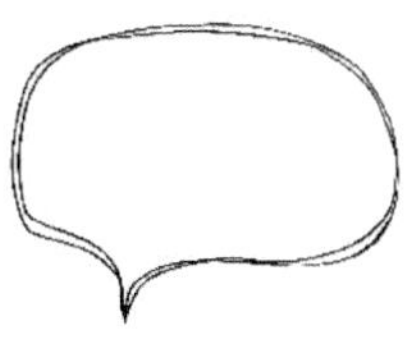

My son has completed SLIT for both environmental and food allergies. I'll share part of that journey here, and more in later sections of the book. Our first experience with SLIT was for environmental allergies when we began OIT treatment for food allergies, something we hadn't planned for or expected.

When I look back, I can see how narrowly focused we were. Compared to managing food allergies, environmental allergies felt like background noise. In reality, they impacted our lives in big and little ways, and were so easy to treat.

AMANDA R. DeSIO WHITEHOUSE, PH.D.

Anaphylactic to Dogs

My son's dog allergy announced itself in a way that was impossible to ignore. He was prone to sniffles and eczema from birth. We didn't notice a significant change in those symptoms when he was around dogs until one visit when a dog licked him on the face. He immediately began to sneeze, develop a rash, and get sniffly. This seemed to calm down until the dog licked him again. After that, the hives spread, his lips, ears, and eyes puffed up, and he became lethargic. It was terrifying, and yet I didn't think to treat it with allergy medications because I didn't realize it could be dangerous. His food allergies weren't diagnosed yet, so I didn't carry emergency medications and wouldn't have known to administer them if we did. We retraced the incident to see if the dog had eaten a food he could be allergic to, but I just didn't know that someone could be *that* allergic to a dog.

When he was diagnosed with food allergies several months later, we discussed the reaction to the dog with the new doctor. She told us to use epinephrine if a reaction that severe occurred again, even to a dog. The guilt and fear of not realizing how severe it had been weighed heavily on me, and moving forward so did the avoidance.

The Quiet Grief of Avoidance

None of our extended family lives locally. Avoiding dogs meant avoiding most family gatherings. We tried to make it work by keeping him in separate rooms and asking that dogs be contained, but more than once we had to pack up and leave early when the hives and facial swelling returned or he started wheezing.

Visits became fewer and farther in between, and there were holidays and traditions we stopped attending because they were hosted in homes where dogs lived or visited along with the rest of the family. It was isolating to feel that our son's health needs unintentionally placed us on the outside of cherished traditions and the new family and holiday memories I'd looked forward to creating for my kids.

Rehoming Our Cat

The dog avoidance was difficult, but not as heartbreaking for me as being advised by our allergist to rehome our sweet black cat, Dewey. Thankfully, one of my closest friends and her husband adored him and spoiled him more than he ever had been at our house. Being able to visit him and see how happy he was softened the blow. But the toll the allergies were quickly taking on all aspects of our lives was difficult to manage.

Starting SLIT: Surprisingly Simple

It wasn't until years later when his environmental allergies were suspected to be impacting his early response to oral immunotherapy (OIT) that our allergist suggested we begin sublingual immunotherapy (SLIT) for environmental allergens. We added the drops during an OIT updose appointment and took the bottle home. Initially, my son developed what he called "the stupid tongue itch" for about 10 minutes after taking the drops. It was annoying but mild and subsided over time, and he never experienced any other symptoms.

By the time his first spring on SLIT rolled around, he was significantly less reactive outdoors during high pollen season. The constant sniffle faded and the itchy eyes and throat clearing diminished. We only used oral antihistamines a handful of times that year.

After several years on SLIT, my son could pet dogs without immediately developing itchy skin, watery eyes, or nasal symptoms. We can even visit homes with cats and dogs without issue now. He still washes his hands and changes clothes when he gets home, but he tolerates being there comfortably.

He has now been off the drops for almost two years and has maintained his tolerance, and a recent skin test was negative to dogs. If symptoms re-emerge, we would restart treatment without hesitation to boost his tolerance. This aspect of his immunotherapy journey alone was so impactful by helping us regain flexibility and access to our community.

The Costs and Gains

The downside of SLIT was that insurance did not cover the cost. Initially, when the drops were mixed in our allergist's office, the cost was reasonable, but when the doctor began to outsource to an outside manufacturer and pricing structures changed, the cost rose significantly. Eventually, we transitioned care to another allergy practice that was able to order the drops from the outside manufacturer and provide them at cost. We would invest in them again if needed, but the variation in cost over the years has been significant.

When I consider the benefits of environmental SLIT, the cost was well-worth it. It reduced the daily inflammatory burden on his body and supported his OIT journey. Over time, it softened social barriers and allowed my son to be included in new ways.

Biologic Medications

In recent years, biologic medications have reshaped the conversation about what is possible in food allergy care. On episode 86 of the *Don't Feed the Fear* podcast, Dr. Brian Vickery discussed the science and its rapid pace of change in this area (Whitehouse & Vickery, 2026). Dr. Vickery is Vice Chair of Clinical Research for the Emory School of Medicine Department of Pediatrics, Division Chief of Allergy and Immunology, and Director of the Food Allergy Program at Children's Healthcare of Atlanta. He is a nationally recognized leader in advancing evidence-based therapies for food allergy and anaphylaxis.

A biologic is a type of medication made from antibodies. Antibodies are proteins our immune systems naturally produce to fight infection and regulate immune responses. Over the past two decades, researchers have learned how to engineer antibodies into medicines that target very specific parts of the immune system. Unlike older medications that can affect many systems in the body at once, biologics are designed to act in a very precise way rather than affecting the whole system. They are highly targeted, binding to one specific molecule or pathway.

That precision is one of their greatest strengths. Because biologic medications act only on what they are designed to recognize, they don't cause the broad systemic side effects that can accompany other classes of drugs. In allergy, that means targeting the allergic arm of the immune system while leaving the rest of the immune defenses largely intact (Whitehouse & Vickery, 2026).

Omalizumab and the Approval of a Biologic for Food Allergy

In February 2024, omalizumab, known by the brand name Xolair, became the first biologic approved by the FDA for the treatment of food allergy. According to Dr. Vickery, omalizumab had already been in use for nearly twenty years for asthma and chronic hives, but its approval for food allergy marked a major turning point (Whitehouse & Vickery, 2026).

Omalizumab works by binding to IgE, the antibody central to allergic reactions. By attaching to circulating IgE and preventing it from triggering allergic cells, omalizumab lowers the intensity of the allergic response. In a large study called the Omalizumab as Monotherapy and as Adjunct Therapy in Children and Adults with Food Allergy or "OUTMATCH" trial, four months of omalizumab treatment significantly increased the amount of allergenic food patients could tolerate and reduced reaction risk across multiple food allergies, supporting its role as a protective (but not curative) therapy (Wood et al., 2024). For many, that translates into meaningful protection from accidental exposures.

Dr. Vickery shared that one of the most important features of omalizumab is that its effect is not food specific. Unlike oral immunotherapy, which targets only the foods treated, omalizumab can increase tolerance across all allergens. This is particularly relevant for the thirty to forty percent of patients who live with more than one food allergy. It is also approved for use starting at age one and extends into adulthood (Whitehouse & Vickery, 2026).

Dupilumab for Eczema, Asthma, and EoE

Another biologic medication relevant to the allergy community is dupilumab, marketed as Dupixent. Dupilumab is approved for moderate to severe eczema, asthma, and eosinophilic esophagitis (EoE), all of which are chronic allergic diseases. It works by blocking a key inflammatory signal in the allergic pathway. By interrupting that signal, IgE levels in the blood decrease (Tian et al, 2025; Zaazouee et al., 2022).

While Dupixent lowers IgE levels, this reduction does not reliably translate into increased food tolerance in older children with established allergies. A six-month trial in peanut allergic children demonstrated a significant drop in IgE levels but no meaningful change in reactivity when the food was eaten. For that reason, dupilumab alone is not considered an effective treatment for food allergy (Sindher et al., 2024).

For patients whose primary struggle is uncontrolled eczema or asthma, dupilumab may not change the food allergy itself, but it can dramatically improve overall quality of life by calming other allergic diseases. Dr. Vickery noted that some patients may benefit from a combination of omalizumab and dupilumab. There is no medical contraindication to using them together, though insurance coverage, cost, and the discomfort of injections remain important considerations (Whitehouse & Vickery, 2026).

Biologics in Combination With Immunotherapy

Some patients choose to combine biologics with immunotherapy to reduce the risk of side effects and/or use the medication short-term rather than indefinitely. Dr. Vickery reported that some prefer to calm the immune system with omalizumab, begin OIT while the allergic response is dampened, then discontinue omalizumab once the maintenance dose is reached and tolerated.

Dr. Vickery described omalizumab as an enhanced safety system. It does not fundamentally retrain the immune system because no allergen is introduced, but it reduces the consequences if exposure occurs. OIT, in contrast, changes the immune response to a specific food over time. Some patients prefer one approach over the other. Others pursue both, depending on goals, age, number of allergens, and tolerance for daily dosing (Whitehouse & Vickery, 2026).

The Reality of Ongoing Treatment

One important consideration is that biologics are not curative. When treatment stops, the medication washes out of the system and the protective effect diminishes. For now, families considering biologics must approach them with the understanding that they may represent long term therapy. Dr. Vickery shared an approach that encourages patients and families not to project decades into the future. The field is evolving quickly, next generation medications are already in development, and these may change the options available in the near future (Whitehouse & Vickery, 2026). The pace of change can be both exciting and overwhelming. Increased options means more nuanced decisions.

Safety and Practical Considerations

Omalizumab carries a black box warning for anaphylaxis to the medication itself. Dr. Vickery pointed out that the risk is low, estimated at roughly one in one thousand patients, and most cases occur within the first few doses. For this reason, the first three injections are administered in a clinical setting. After that, patients and families are trained to administer injections at home. The most common side effect is injection site discomfort. The medication is relatively viscous and can sting as it is delivered. Doses vary, and most patients require injections every two to four weeks to reach their target amount (Whitehouse & Vickery, 2026).

Financial considerations are also significant. Even when insurance covers the medication, out of pocket costs may be substantial. Biologics offer meaningful advances, and require thoughtful, individualized decision-making grounded in medical facts, family goals, and practical realities.

Choosing Possibility in the Midst of Uncertainty

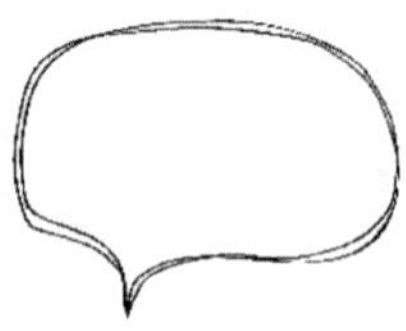

Mia Silverman didn't set out to become a voice for the food allergy community. It started with one video during the early days of COVID lockdown: a lighthearted clip listing some of her allergies set to a quirky song. She posted it without much thought. By the next day, it had nearly a million views.

What began as a moment of connection quickly grew into a platform where she shared the realities of living with over 50 food allergies on her social media platform, @allergieswithmia. She is known for showing the logistics of allergy life and the lived experience behind them.

Living With Anxiety and Moving Forward Anyway

Mia has multiple allergies and a long history of severe reactions since childhood. While she has outgrown a small number of her allergens, the reality of living with dozens of allergens has meant constant vigilance. Every meal, every restaurant, every social event requires planning and awareness. Even something as small as cross-contact can carry significant risk.

With so many allergens, avoidance isn't simple. The world isn't designed for that level of sensitivity, and that reality brings an ongoing baseline of anxiety. For most of her life, Mia was told that food allergy treatments weren't an option for her because her allergies were too severe. When she first heard a different perspective that treatment might actually be possible, her instinct was skepticism. It felt too different from everything she had been told.

Reconsidering What's Possible

At an allergy advocacy event, Mia learned more about treatment options and had discussions that felt encouraging and possibility-focused rather than centered only on limitations. Instead of being told what could not be done or how rare her case was, she was introduced to the idea that treatment might be worth exploring.

This new perspective led her to seek out a new provider whose approach felt more collaborative, hopeful, and forward-thinking. She took time to research, ask questions, and talk to others who had gone through similar therapies. She considered the success stories and also the challenges of immunotherapy such as daily exposure to allergens, consistency over time, and the ability to cope with discomfort, possible symptoms/reactions, and uncertainty.

Rather than rushing into a decision, Mia gave herself space to fully understand what treatment would require and whether it aligned with her goals, her capacity, and the life she wanted to build.

Holding Fear and Hope at the Same Time

After discussing her options with her new doctor, Mia decided to begin omalizumab treatments to reduce reactivity, then move forward with OIT for peanuts, sesame, cashew, and milk. Mia has opted not to treat her salmon allergy, because she notes it is easy to avoid and she isn't interested in dosing that food on a daily basis. She was prescribed omalizumab in the past, tolerated it well, and experienced no food allergy reactions during the time she was taking the medication. Prior to that, she had frequent accidental exposures and reactions. Though she dislikes needles, Mia said that tolerating the shot as she began treatment again is worth it given her hope of treatment success.

Ultimately, Mia made her decision to pursue combined omalizumab and OIT treatment with an open mind, expecting both anxiety and hope to coexist. Mia feels empowered by the powerful study showing that it is helpful for OIT patients to frame symptoms as positive signals (sometimes abbreviated the "SAPS" approach; Howe et al., 2019), and is moving forward with treatment viewing potential symptoms as an indication that her body may be adapting. She hopes this mindset will allow her to stay engaged, even during difficult times.

Defining Her Own Goals

For Mia, the goal isn't a cure or even incorporating her allergens regularly into her diet. For her, the treatment and all it entails will be worth it if she can eat safely at a restaurant without constant risk and fear of cross-contact. Her goal is having more ease and less mental load in everyday moments.

As she moves forward, Mia continues to share her experience openly in hopes of spreading the word that there might be options even for the most severe patients who thought they weren't possible. Find her on social media @allergieswithmia to follow her immunotherapy journey in the years ahead.

Explaining Biologics to Children

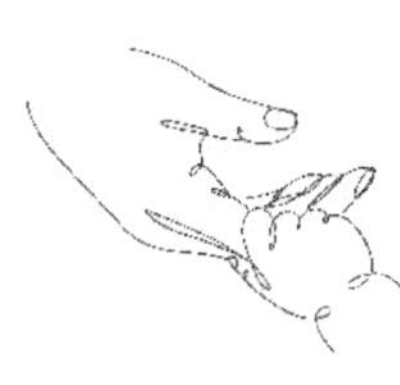

Biologics are a type of medicine that helps your immune system not to have such a big reaction to allergens. They are given as shots at the clinic or sometimes at home. They don't cure allergies, but they can help to decrease symptoms like hives, asthma, EoE, and the likelihood of an allergic reaction depending on which one is chosen. Be sure to clarify what symptoms the biologic medication you are choosing can help with, since they each have different target symptoms.

Under 5: Concrete, Simple, and Reassuring

Young children focus on immediate experiences and need short, literal explanations.

You might say:
"This medicine helps your body with allergies. It might pinch for a second, and we will plan ways to deal with that."

Helpful strategies:

- Use simple words like "poke."
- Keep the routine predictable: "We go, get the poke, read and snack while we wait, then go home."
- Provide comfort: hold their hand, offer a favorite toy or security item
- Focus on small, achievable goals: "We do one shot at a time."

Ages 5-8: Building Understanding and Mastery

Children in early elementary school can understand cause-and-effect and like to be involved.

You might say:
"This medicine can help your immune system and can help with allergy symptoms. We give it as a shot at the doctor's office at first, and eventually we might be able to take it at home."

Helpful strategies:

- Offer choices when possible about any aspect of the day (snacks, toys, comfort measures)
- Normalize feelings: it's okay to feel nervous about shots and excited about improvement.
- Connect to daily life: explain how it may make playground, school, or meals easier.
- Give them a sense of control: "You are helping protect your body."

Ages 9–12: More Detail and Collaborative Framing

Older children can understand nuances, schedules, and safety monitoring.

You might say:
"Biologics are medicines that help your immune system stop overreacting. You get them as shots and over time, your symptoms might decrease. For extra safety, we do it at the doctor's office at first."

Helpful strategies:

- Explain dosing schedules and clinic check-ins.
- Prepare them for mild reactions at home (like redness or itchiness at the injection site).
- Invite them to share concerns or questions.
- Emphasize progress as a journey, not perfection: "Each shot is a step toward feeling better."

Teens: Transparency, Autonomy, and Goal-Oriented Framing

Adolescents benefit from direct discussion of risks, benefits, and long-term goals.

You might say:
"Biologics are medicines that help your immune system be less reactive to allergens, and can decrease your symptoms. Shots are given on a regular schedule and most reactions are mild. At first they are given at the doctor's office, and can eventually be given at home."

Helpful strategies:

- Engage them in planning: when to schedule shots, how to monitor responses.

- Discuss realistic expectations: biologics reduce reactions but do not cure allergies, they may be used in conjunction with OIT to decrease reactivity to doses.

- Validate feelings: nervousness, excitement, or frustration are normal.

- Connect the treatment to personal goals: improved freedom, safety, and confidence.

Emerging or Experimental Treatments

Traditional Chinese Medicine for Eczema and Food Allergies

Dr. Xiu-Min Li is a clinician and researcher who has pioneered the use of Traditional Chinese Medicine (TCM) in the context of Western medical practices to treat severe eczema and food allergies. In episode 95 of the *Don't Feed the Fear* podcast, Dr. Li explained that she trained in both Eastern and Western medicine, allowing her to combine the holistic principles of TCM with evidence-based research methods, including clinical trials and biomarker analysis. Her approach emphasizes supporting the whole body, gradually restoring balance, and modulating immune responses rather than simply suppressing symptoms (Whitehouse & Li, 2026).

Dr. Li said, "We know that TCM works. Our job is to find out why it works and how to make it work better." In her privately operated clinic, her patients' treatment protocols include some combination of herbal baths, creams, oral herbal teas, and capsules, as well as acupuncture and acupressure. Progress is monitored using both clinical outcomes and objective biomarkers, such as skin integrity and immunologic assays. Families interested in TCM can work directly with Dr. Li at her integrative medicine center in Mamaronek, in collaboration with family allergists and pediatricians to ensure safety and effectiveness (Whitehouse & Li, 2026).

Clinical Integration and Research

Dr. Li's food allergy herbal formula (FAHF-2) showed promise for food allergy and immune modulation in laboratory studies and animal models (Wang et al., 2015). Dr. Li and her team subsequently identified berberine as the key active component of FAHF-2. However, it had a crucial drawback–lack of bioavailability, meaning that it passed through the body too rapidly to achieve therapeutic efficacy. Isolated and refined through use of a nano particle, berberine has been shown to lower production of the allergic antibody while preserving overall immune health (Yang et al., 2014).

TCM targets multiple aspects of immune function simultaneously, aiming for sustainable improvement rather than temporary symptom control. Dr. Li said she envisions therapies that could provide long-lasting relief, not just temporary symptom management, with the potential to fundamentally reset the immune system and improve quality of life for patients with multiple allergic conditions. Her ongoing clinical and laboratory work aims to make these approaches safer, more effective, and widely accessible, offering hope to families navigating the challenges of food allergies, asthma, severe eczema, and other immune disorders (Whitehouse & Li, 2026).

Our Experience with Traditional Chinese Medicine

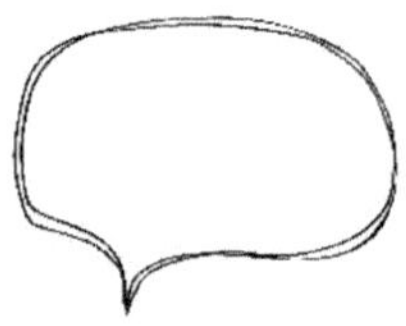

After my son was initially diagnosed, I was drawn to holistic treatment options and found Traditional Chinese Medicine (TCM). Its goal is to address underlying immune imbalance rather than just manage symptoms.

Fear, Protection, and Choice

The idea of healing my son without direct allergen exposure aligned with my instinct to protect him while honoring the body as an integrated system. What I read about Dr. Li's perspective also mirrored what I was learning about the nervous system's role in immune function and resilience. I'd read about OIT, but my doctors told me it was dangerous and it wasn't available anyway. They were wrong, their comments led me to pursue TCM, which offered what I hoped would be a gentle, holistic path.

Commitment and Challenges

Getting onto Dr. Li's clinic schedule required navigating skepticism from my local doctors, additional testing, a waitlist, and the daunting stress of traveling with food allergies. I tried to create meaningful rituals, like making an "allergy buddy" stuffed animal at *Build-A-Bear*, to help him feel safe. We even got his buddy a matching allergy alert bracelet. These comfort items would end up carrying forward as a comforting constant even when we eventually changed treatments. The daily protocol was demanding for a 4-year-old child: medicinal bath soaks, thick cream application, and bitter herbs consumed. The significant time and energy required were compounded by caring for three boys ages 4 and under.

Progress and Transition

My son's compliance was remarkable, but the regimen and cost became increasingly difficult for us all to sustain. When the opportunity arose to join the peanut patch clinical trial, it was clear that it was time to try a different path. We discontinued TCM with gratitude and without regret, maintaining respect for the work that had shaped his care and the chance to be part of this emerging treatment, which I still believe will eventually lead to breakthroughs in eczema and allergy care.

This experience recalibrated my sense of what was possible and informed every treatment decision that followed. Even though this path wasn't sustainable for us long-term, it made future treatments feel more manageable and strengthened my resolve.

Epicutaneous Immunotherapy (EPIT)

The "peanut patch," also known as epicutaneous immunotherapy (EPIT), is an emerging treatment designed to help reduce the risk of severe reactions to peanut exposure. The patch (brand name *Viaskin*) is worn on the skin daily and delivers a very small amount of peanut protein through the skin rather than by mouth. Over time, this consistent exposure aims to retrain the immune system and increase tolerance to peanut. The peanut patch is currently in late-stage clinical development with potential market availability in the near future if approved. A milk patch is also in development, though not as far along in the approval process at this time.

What the Research Shows

Clinical trials suggest that the peanut patch can increase the amount of peanut protein a child can tolerate, which may help protect against severe reactions from accidental exposure. A significantly higher percentage of children using the patch met treatment response criteria compared to placebo, and most side effects have been mild and localized to the skin, such as irritation at the patch site, with low rates of systemic reactions (Greenhawt et al., 2025). While peanut EPIT is the most advanced, studies are underway for other food allergens.

Where It May Fit in the Treatment Landscape

If approved, the peanut patch may offer a less invasive, lower-risk alternative to oral immunotherapy (OIT), especially for younger children or families who find daily ingestion stressful or difficult to maintain. Rather than aiming for full tolerance, the patch is best understood as a way to reduce risk and increase safety in real-world situations, particularly accidental exposures. It may become an important option within a broader, individualized treatment plan that could include avoidance, emergency preparedness, and other therapies.

Our Experience With the Peanut Patch

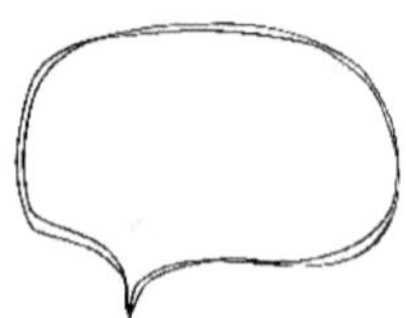

After my son's experience with traditional Chinese medicine for allergies, we found a clinical trial for the peanut patch. For a highly sensitive and reactive child, epicutaneous exposure felt gentler than ingestion, and participating in research was meaningful and accessible.

The staff at our trial site were wonderful and trial participation had its perks, including free treatment and reimbursement for some of our travel expenses. The patch itself turned out to be more challenging than expected. My son tolerated wearing it, but the skin irritation from the allergen on the skin and the adhesive were very uncomfortable for him. Following the strict trial protocol added extra demands: lack of personalization of care, documenting reactions carefully, and communicating with the research team.

The trial instructions required the patch to be rotated between six specific spots on the back. When it came time to rotate back to the initial application site and apply a new patch, my son's skin in that spot was still broken and irritated. I called the clinic staff, and they instructed me to apply to the first application site regardless of the condition of his skin. As we drove to the research center, my son began coughing. He hadn't been sick so it seemed strange, and I grew increasingly concerned as I drove and the cough worsened.

It wasn't until we arrived and I removed his hat and saw the hives on his neck that I realized what was happening. I rushed him inside and asked staff to administer epinephrine, and once they did the reaction immediately subsided. After that, we obtained permission to use a broader range of sites on his back to avoid broken skin, and had no more issues. We continued for a time but ultimately transitioned to a private OIT provider for a more individualized approach.

Looking back, I would administer epinephrine sooner, but otherwise, I am glad we tried the patch. It may have helped him gain some tolerance that made OIT go more smoothly, though of course we'll never know for certain. What stayed with me most was how the experience sharpened my ability to recognize risk, manage uncertainty, and advocate for my son's individual needs.

I am not sharing this story to criticize any treatment, but to be honest and realistic. It is my hope that his story provides encouragement that even a child as sensitive as mine can progress successfully through treatment, even if it requires navigating the options available and finding the path that works best for them.

Intralymphatic Immunotherapy (ILIT) for Environmental Allergies

Intralymphatic immunotherapy, or ILIT, is an emerging treatment for environmental allergies (not foods) that works slightly differently from traditional allergy shots or sublingual immunotherapy (SLIT) drops. Instead of weekly or monthly injections over several years, ILIT delivers small amounts of allergen directly into a lymph node using a carefully guided needle over fewer sessions to teach the immune system to tolerate environmental allergens.

How It Works

Dr. Kara Wada provides ILIT in her practice, and described the procedure in episode 87 of the *Don't Feed the Fear* podcast. Dr. Wada is a board-certified allergist and immunologist specializing in complex immune conditions, including Mast Cell Activation Syndrome (MCAS), Sjögren's Disease, and other autoimmune diseases. She shares her integrative, patient-centered and personal experience-informed approach through multiple podcasts, including the *Becoming Immune Confident Podcast*, and her social media account @immuneconfidentmd.

According to Dr. Wada, ILIT is done under careful supervision with ultrasound guidance to ensure the needle reaches the lymph node before the allergen is injected. Most patients report little discomfort beyond the initial pinch, though some may experience temporary swelling or itching at the injection site. Patients are monitored for systemic reactions, and they always bring their epinephrine device as a precaution (Whitehouse & Wada, 2026). Compared to allergy shots (SCIT), ILIT carries a significantly lower risk of a systemic reaction and requires far fewer injections (Wang et al., 2023).

Timing and Effectiveness

Patients usually receive three injections spaced four weeks apart. Initial improvements in symptoms, like reduced sneezing, congestion, or asthma flare-ups, often become noticeable after the second or third visit. For seasonal allergies, ILIT can sometimes be timed so that the treatment concludes just as allergy season begins, helping patients experience relief when they need it most. Individuals who have struggled with traditional immunotherapy or who have busy schedules may find ILIT particularly appealing (Whitehouse & Wada, 2026).

Who It's For

ILIT is typically recommended for adults and older children, usually around 6–7 years and up, depending on size, maturity, and comfort with needles. Those who want a shorter, more targeted treatment course often consider ILIT as an alternative to weekly shots or daily SLIT drops (Whitehouse & Wada, 2026). While ILIT is not yet widely offered, it represents an exciting option and area for future growth in the allergy treatment landscape.

Future Directions

The landscape of food allergy treatment is expanding rapidly, offering new options beyond avoidance and emergency epinephrine. Additional medications and allergen-specific vaccines and next-generation immunotherapies are under investigation, our understanding are being developed. Researchers and clinicians are actively pursuing treatments that may reduce reactions, improve quality of life, and even move us closer to ending food allergies.

Considering Eosinophilic Esophagitis (EoE)

 When families begin exploring immunotherapy for food allergies, one term that often appears in conversations is Eosinophilic Esophagitis (pronounced EE-oh-sin-uh-FIL-ik eh-SOF-a-JII-tis) or EoE. In the food allergy community, EoE is frequently discussed and sometimes feared, particularly in relation to treatments that require swallowing allergens. Understanding what EoE is and how it differs from other allergic conditions can help families make decisions that are more informed and less fear-driven.

Dr. Christopher Parrish addressed EoE in the context of OIT in episode 84 of the *Don't Feed the Fear* podcast (Whitehouse & Parrish, 2026). Dr. Parrish is triple board certified in allergy and clinical immunology, pediatrics, and internal medicine. He currently leads Latitude Food Allergy Care's Orange County Clinic in Irvine, California, where he provides specialized care for food allergy patients of all ages. Prior to his current role, Dr. Parrish was an investigator in clinical trials for food allergy and eosinophilic esophagitis (EoE) which led to the first FDA-approved therapies for each of these conditions, and founded a multidisciplinary clinic for children with EoE and other forms of eosinophilic gastrointestinal disorders.

What is EoE?

EoE is a chronic allergic inflammatory condition of the esophagus, the tube that carries food from the mouth to the stomach. Dr. Parrish explained EoE by comparing it to eczema. In eczema, the skin barrier is not functioning properly, allowing irritants and allergens to trigger inflammation on the surface of the skin. In EoE, the lining of the esophagus does not form as strong a protective barrier as it should, allowing food proteins to interact with the immune system and trigger allergic-type inflammation in the esophageal tissue (Whitehouse & Parrish, 2026).

EoE Symptoms

Dr. Parrish noted that the symptoms of EoE can look very different depending on a person's age. In adolescents and adults, the most common symptom is difficulty swallowing, particularly with dense foods like meat or bread. Food may feel like it gets stuck in the chest while going down. Sometimes a person needs to drink water to help food pass. In more severe cases, food can become lodged in the esophagus and require medical attention to remove it.

In younger children, the symptoms can be much less specific. Infants and toddlers may experience frequent vomiting that seems random rather than tied to a specific food. Some children develop feeding difficulties or strong preferences for soft foods like yogurt or purees. They may avoid chunky textures or struggle to transition to solid foods. According to Dr. Parrish, these challenges can affect growth if eating becomes too uncomfortable.

Because these symptoms overlap with many other childhood experiences, EoE can be difficult to recognize. Diagnosis requires an endoscopy with biopsy, a procedure that allows doctors to look at the esophagus and examine a tissue sample under a microscope to count eosinophils and confirm inflammation (Whitehouse & Parrish, 2026).

Treatment Options

Dr. Parrish shared several EoE treatment approaches that may be considered. One option is dietary therapy, which involves removing foods from the diet that are suspected to be triggering inflammation. Unlike IgE-mediated allergies, traditional allergy testing does not reliably identify EoE triggers. Instead, doctors often use a stepwise elimination approach, removing common trigger foods such as dairy or wheat and then monitoring whether inflammation improves.

Another option involves medications that reduce inflammation in the esophagus. These can include proton pump inhibitors (acid-reducing medications that also have anti-inflammatory effects), swallowed topical steroids that coat the esophagus, or the biologic medications dupilumab that targets specific immune pathways involved in allergic inflammation. While EoE is considered a chronic condition, it is also manageable, and many people find effective ways to control symptoms and maintain a good quality of life (Whitehouse & Parrish, 2026).

Weighing Risks and Benefits

For families considering immunotherapy for food allergies, one of the most common concerns is whether treatments like OIT could trigger EoE. Studies show that the overall risk of EoE during or after OIT is relatively low, but do support careful monitoring for EoE symptoms during treatment (Lucendo et al., 2014). A more recent analysis of children undergoing OIT revealed that fewer than 1% developed new-onset EoE during OIT (Buckey et al., 2026). In other words, the vast majority of people undergoing OIT do not develop EoE.

Dr. Parrish clarified that if EoE does occur during immunotherapy, it does not automatically mean that treatment must stop. In many cases, families and physicians work together to explore different options. Some may adjust dosing, slow the treatment process, switch to SLIT which does not require swallowing the allergens, or treat the EoE while continuing immunotherapy. These decisions often involve careful discussions about risks, benefits, and each family's priorities.

One perspective Dr. Parrish's patients sometimes consider is that food allergies can carry the risk of life-threatening anaphylaxis, while EoE is not life-threatening even though it can affect quality of life. For some families, this changes how they think about the trade-offs involved in treatment decisions (Whitehouse & Parrish, 2026).

Ultimately, these choices are deeply personal. Every patient and family brings their own experiences, fears, and goals to the table. Learning about conditions like EoE can help shift the conversation from one driven primarily by fear to one guided by information, perspective, and thoughtful decision-making.

EoE Fears

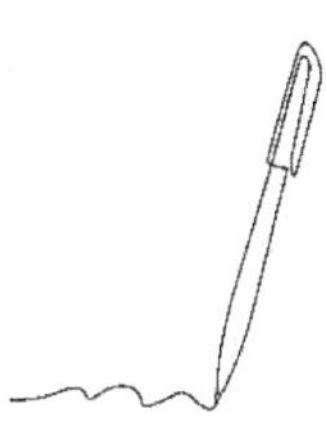

This worksheet is for those who do not have EoE, but worry about the possibility of developing Eosinophilic Esophagitis (EoE) due to treatment. It can be helpful to slow down and separate our fears from the information we actually have. *It is recommended that you skip this page if this is not a concern for you. If you have EoE, move ahead to the worksheet on the next page.*

Name the Worry

Write down the thoughts or worries that come up when you think about immunotherapy and EoE.

____

____

What Do I Know?

Write down the facts you learned about EoE from your doctor, reliable research, and this book.

____

____

Challenge the Thought

Address the worries with the following questions:

My worry:

____

____

Evidence that supports this worry:

____

____

Evidence that does not support this worry:

____

____

A more balanced way to think about this:

____

____

What Would Help Me Feel More Informed?

Write down questions or concerns you want to discuss with your medical team

____

____

____

Thinking Through EoE and Immunotherapy

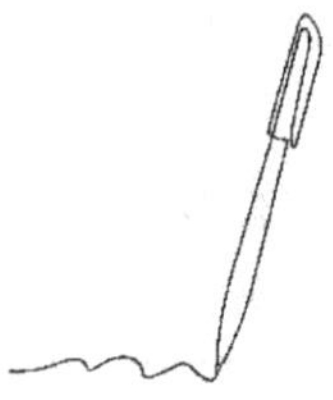

If you or your child has been diagnosed with Eosinophilic Esophagitis, or your doctor suspects it may be present, there may be decisions to make about how to proceed with treatment. Some patients with EoE decide to begin or continue OIT with the support of their medical team. This worksheet helps you weigh the potential benefits and risks in a way that reflects your own priorities.

Use this to think through your thoughts and questions prior to an appointment and to take notes during your discussion with your provider.

My Experience

What symptoms or experiences with EoE have I managed, and what impact have they had?

____

____

____

Medical Information I Have So Far

Diagnosis status:　　☐ Confirmed EoE　　☐ Suspected EoE　　☐ Being evaluated/monitored

Questions for my doctor about symptoms, tests, and diagnosis:

____

____

____

Potential Benefits of Treatment Options

☐ Increased protection against accidental exposures　　☐ Reduced risk of severe allergic reactions

☐ Reduced anxiety about accidental ingestion　　☐ Greater flexibility with food choices

☐ Participate in experiences previously avoided　　☐ Improved quality of life

☐ Possibility of desensitization or tolerance　　☐ Reduced burden of strict avoidance

☐ Ease in daily functioning (school/work, travel)　　☐ Increased independence

Other reasons or thoughts about these:

____

____

____

____

Concerns or Barriers

What concerns or barriers do you have about beginning/continuing immunotherapy with EoE?

☐ Concern with worsening EoE symptoms ☐ Risk of triggering new esophageal inflammation

☐ Need for ongoing monitoring ☐ Potential need for endoscopy or additional testing

☐ Increased medical appointments ☐ Time commitment for dosing and clinic visits

☐ Managing symptoms that may occur ☐ Uncertainty about how the body will respond

☐ Emotional stress associated with daily exposure to an allergen

Other concerns and thoughts/notes:

____
____
____
____

Questions for Our Medical Team

☐ Do you recommend treatment, and if so which one(s)?
☐ How does EoE affect immunotherapy decisions in our case?
☐ What symptoms should we watch for and how will we monitor for them?
☐ How would we monitor for changes in EoE?
☐ What would cause us to pause, adjust, or stop treatment?

____
____
____
____

Our Values and Priorities

When making decisions about treatment, what is important to you?

☐ EoE symptom relief ☐ Mental Health/Less Anxiety ☐ Safety
☐ Minimizing medical procedures ☐ Long-term outcomes ☐ Quality of life

Other values and priorities and notes about these:

____
____
____

Decision Balance Scale

Use the scale below to reflect on how the potential benefits and concerns feel to you right now.

1 — 2 — 3 — 4 — 5 — 6 — 7 — 8 — 9 — 10

Concerns Feel Much Greater   Benefits Feel Much Greater

Building Confidence in Our Decision

Sometimes confidence comes not from having all the answers, but from knowing what would help me feel more prepared to decide.

What additional information, support, or reassurance would help me feel more confident about the path forward?

____

____

____

____

If I decide to move forward or to wait, what signs would tell me that this decision is working well?

____

____

____

____

Next Steps

After considering the information above, what next steps feel reasonable?

☐ Pursue further evaluation   ☐ Seek a second opinion

☐ Gather more information before deciding   ☐ Move forward with treatment planning

☐ Wait and revisit the decision later

Notes or reflections:

____

____

____

____

____

Choosing Not to Pursue Treatment

There is a quiet pressure that many feel as new treatment options are becoming available. When you learn about immunotherapy, biologics, or other approaches, it can begin to feel as though doing something is the "right" choice, and doing nothing is falling behind. That is not an accurate reflection of what thoughtful, informed decision-making looks like in the context of food allergies.

Choosing not to pursue treatment at this time can be a deeply intentional, well-informed, and appropriate decision. For some individuals and families, current medical management feels effective and sustainable. For others, the logistical, emotional, financial, or medical demands of treatment do not align with their current capacity or priorities. In many cases, it is not a matter of whether treatment is "good" or "bad," but whether it is the right fit right now.

It is also important to recognize that timing matters. What feels overwhelming or unmanageable at one stage of life may feel entirely different at another. A young child, a busy family season, co-occurring medical needs, or emotional readiness can all influence the decision. Stepping back is not the same as closing the door. It is often a way of preserving stability while keeping options open for the future.

There can also be emotional complexity in this decision. Some individuals feel relief when they decide not to pursue treatment. Others feel doubt, guilt, or worry about whether they are "doing enough." These reactions are understandable, especially in a culture that often equates action with protection. It may be helpful to remember that thoughtful restraint is also a form of care.

Avoidance and carrying epinephrine has always been, and continues to be, a valid and medically appropriate approach to managing food allergies. Many people with food allergies live full, meaningful lives using this strategy. The goal of this book is not to move you toward treatment, but to support you in making a decision that feels informed, grounded, and aligned with your values.

If you choose not to pursue treatment at this time, the most important outcome is not the decision itself, but how you feel within it. Confidence, clarity, and a sense of peace matter. You deserve to feel settled in your choice, not second-guessing it at every turn.

At the same time, it can be helpful to hold decisions with some flexibility. You may choose to revisit this conversation if circumstances change, if new treatments become available, or if your needs and priorities shift. This is not a one-time decision you must get "right" forever. It is part of an ongoing process of caring for yourself or your child over time.

Choosing "Not Now"

Ina Chung, known for her advocacy on social media through her account @theasianallergymom, has been careful not to let pressure or urgency set the tone for treatment consideration. Her daughter, now eight, has lived with allergies to peanut, dairy, and egg since infancy. Ina has focused her parenting and her advocacy work on reducing the fear around food allergies with education and informed decision-making.

Like many, their family story held more than allergies. With an older son who is neurodivergent, much of their parenting energy was already devoted to creating safety, predictability, and emotional stability at home. Ina describes having a "narrow bandwidth" during those early years, a reality that shaped what was possible.

They focused on living well. Their daughter grew up going to restaurants, attending social events, and navigating her world with thoughtful precautions. There were substitutes, backup plans, caution, and also joy. For a long time, treatment wasn't a question because life felt full and safe as it was.

Planting Seeds, Not Pressure

The shift toward considering treatment came from Ina's daughter, who began around age six to voice sadness about not being able to eat what her friends were having. It wasn't constant, but it was new, and Ina logged that change as important. She responded with gentle introduction, planting seeds about treatments and what changes they could bring.

When her daughter first heard about OIT, the answer was an immediate *no*. Ina accepted that answer and gave her daughter space rather than trying to convince her or reframe the conversation. Over time, the conversation resurfaced in unexpected ways during moments of curiosity, longing, and imagination. A glimpse of her brother's food, a passing comment about what it might be like to try it, and a dream of traveling to Paris and eating freely were some signs that her daughter might be open to revisiting the idea.

Each time, Ina offered information carefully and sparingly, mindful not to overpromise. She described treatment in simple, accurate terms, correcting misconceptions along the way, like her daughter's early belief that OIT meant drinking a glass of milk beginning on the first day of treatment.

Through their gentle conversations, something shifted. The idea of treatment became less abstract, and more connected to her daughter's own desires until one day, she said, "I want to do it." Even then, Ina held it lightly. She scheduled the consultation with the allergist, but remained prepared for her daughter to change her mind.

Holding Reality Alongside Hope

As Ina learned more about treatment options, she noticed that her own hope was growing. She heard stories of children eating previously unsafe foods, the expanding conversations around therapies, the possibility of change, and began to imagine a different future.

Ina had already done the complex work of accepting that her daughter's allergies might be lifelong. That acceptance didn't mean giving up hope. It contextualized the hope, and allowed her to approach treatment as something she could thoughtfully consider without urgency. This mindset became an anchor: *We will be okay either way.*

An Unexpected Turn

By the time they arrived at their consultation, Ina's daughter seemed to be curious and motivated. Ina was surprised when the allergist explained that their clinic did not offer OIT for dairy or egg, the very allergens most impacting her daughter's daily life. Peanut OIT was available, but it wasn't a meaningful priority for her daughter, who finds peanuts easy to avoid.

The doctor suggested omalizumab treatments instead, and her daughter immediately knew that she was not willing to choose a treatment involving shots. The conversation continued, thorough and thoughtful, but the direction was becoming clear. By the end of the appointment, the decision had quietly emerged: *Not now.*

The Wisdom of Declining

There was no dramatic moment or definitive conclusion, but the moment that made the decision clear to Ina was when her tired child spoke her own simple yet powerful truth: "It's okay having my allergy."

Ina felt the weight of that moment as clarity. She felt at peace having asked questions, considered their options, and arriving at a decision that was grounded in her daughter's wants and needs.

Leaving the Door Open

After the appointment, Ina was somewhat disappointed, but returned to what she knew to be true. They had been safely managing the allergies and her daughter was confident and thriving. The decision not to pursue treatment was not closed, but for that moment it was settled.

Perhaps the most defining feature of Ina's approach is not the decision itself, but the way she holds it confidently and without finality. Ina continues to learn more, especially about how effective OIT can be for egg and milk allergies. If changes arise, the conversation will still be there, ready to be revisited. For now, the decision feels informed, regulated, and aligned.

Chapter 2:
Understanding Allergy Anxiety and Trauma

 As you now know, medical research has made remarkable progress in understanding, managing, and even treating food allergies. These advances offer hope for fewer reactions, more flexibility in daily life, and, potentially, a path toward long-term tolerance.

Yet, even with these options, living with food allergies involves far more than medical management. Every meal, social event, or school day can carry uncertainty. Many patients and families experience ongoing anxiety, worry, and stress as they navigate daily life weighing risks and anticipating potential reactions. The burden is not just about physical health. It touches mental and emotional well-being and all aspects of daily life.

Deciding on and following through with treatment can add a mental load that strains an already stretched capacity for focus and decision-making. There are decisions about which therapies to try, how to balance safety with effectiveness, and how to integrate them into busy family or personal schedules. These choices are complicated by questions about long-term outcomes, side effects, and even accessibility. Fear, stress, and second-guessing are common parts of the food allergy experience, and all this spills over into treatment decisions.

Many patients and parents also carry the emotional weight of past reactions. Some have experienced severe allergic episodes or near-misses that leave lasting trauma. Others experience the constant vigilance and anticipatory anxiety even if they have never experienced a severe reaction. These emotional experiences are natural responses to living with a condition that can feel unpredictable and can genuinely be dangerous.

What Makes Food Allergy Anxiety Unique

Living with food allergies brings a type of anxiety unlike most others. A key reason for this is that the physical sensations of anxiety can closely mimic the signs of an allergic reaction. Racing heart, shortness of breath, nausea, and hives can all be very real physiological responses to anxiety, and can create a loop where worry about a reaction triggers physical symptoms, which in turn increase uncertainty and fear.

In contrast to many anxiety presentations, food allergy anxiety reflects a real and ongoing risk, and complete avoidance of the trigger is not always possible. Food is everywhere, and we must eat daily. Most forms of immunotherapy require us to consume or be exposed to the very foods that once caused reactions. This can feel daunting, because the process asks us to engage with both the physical reality of the allergic response and the emotional memory of past reactions.

These layers of body and mind are where the concept of gradual exposure becomes central to navigating food allergies. The concept of exposure therapy is a well-established approach in treating anxiety: by safely and gradually confronting what we fear, we can retrain the nervous system to respond with less panic

(Abramowitz et al., 2019). In food allergy treatment, a similar principle is at play. Immunotherapy provides controlled, incremental exposure to allergens, helping the body develop tolerance. At the same time, exposure therapy techniques can help food allergy patients work through the emotional and psychological barriers to this process (Ramos and Herbert, 2020).

Please note: this workbook is not a substitute for formal exposure and response prevention (ERP) therapy. ERP is a clinical process that should be guided by a trained professional. The concept of gradual exposure will help you recognize the layers of challenge at hand.

Undergoing immunotherapy treatment involves two distinct layers of exposure:

1. Medical exposure: the body's gradual adaptation to the allergen through controlled doses.

2. Emotional exposure: addressing anxiety, trauma, and avoidance behaviors in a safe and supportive way in the context of preparing for and engaging in the treatment.

To be effective, exposure to address anxiety must involve:

- Safety and predictability: the individual must feel supported and know what to expect.

- Gradual progression: small, manageable steps build confidence and tolerance.

- Mind-body awareness: noticing internal sensations, emotions, and patterns of avoidance.

- Response prevention: resisting the urge to escape or avoid, which reinforces fear.

Body-based, somatic, and trauma-informed care are central to this process, particularly to the prevention of responses that can exacerbate rather than decrease anxiety. Understanding and addressing nervous system responses through this process ensures that emotional and physiological challenges are addressed together, without creating more trauma, and with compassion and respect for each person's experience.

The upcoming sections will explore concepts and practical strategies to address and limit anxiety so that it hopefully becomes a manageable part of your journey rather than an overwhelming barrier. For many who pursue treatment, anxiety may feel heightened at first. Over time, however, this investment often leads to increased tolerance, greater safety, and a meaningful reduction in overall anxiety.

Anxiety vs. Trauma in Food Allergies

Anxiety

Anxiety is a natural, future-oriented response to perceived threat. It is the body's way of preparing us to anticipate and prevent danger. In the context of food allergies, anxiety might show up as worry about a possible reaction, heightened vigilance around food, or repeated checking behaviors to ensure safety. Anxiety activates the body's physiological threat response system, often called our "fight or flight" state, leading to symptoms like a racing heart, shallow breathing, nausea, or dizziness. These sensations are not imagined or "in your head." They are real, body-based responses created by the body to help us achieve safety in times of threat or danger (American Psychiatric Association [APA], 2022).

For those with food allergies, this becomes complex because the very real danger of being exposed to the allergens is not effectively managed through an urgent, anxious response. The actions that keep us safe are careful preparation, knowledge, and appropriate caution. Anxiety becomes a threat to our safety as it reduces our capacity for thinking clearly, can lead to rash decisions, or motivates us to avoid situations or experiences beyond what is necessary for safety. For many, anxiety is what prevents them from pursuing a treatment that could increase safety and improve quality of life.

Trauma

Trauma is not about anticipating a future threat. It is the imprint of a past experience that overwhelmed the body's ability to cope at the time. A severe allergic reaction is genuinely life-threatening and can involve rapid symptom escalation, severe symptoms, loss of control, and emergency intervention, all of which can be experienced by the nervous system as traumatic.

Rather than being future-focused like anxiety, trauma is often past-based but felt in the present and often mistaken for a current threat. With little or no conscious thought, the body may respond as though the danger is happening again, even in situations that are objectively safe. This can lead to intense physical and emotional reactions that seem to come "out of nowhere," including panic, shutdown, or a strong urge to escape (Herman, 2015).

From a body-based perspective, trauma is held not just in memory, but in the nervous system. The body learns to associate certain sensations, environments, or experiences with danger, and can react automatically before the "thinking brain" has time to assess what is actually happening (Levine, 2010).

Trauma is not defined only by rare or extreme events. It is defined by how the body and nervous system respond to experiences that feel threatening, overwhelming, or out of control. In the context of food allergies, those experiences can include severe reactions, anaphylaxis, emergency room visits, medical procedures, repeated close calls, or even the ongoing unpredictability of living with a condition that can become life-threatening quickly.

For some, trauma develops from a single intense event. For others, it builds over time through repeated moments of fear, vigilance, and uncertainty. The body learns that the world is not fully safe, and it adapts in ways that are meant to protect, even if those adaptations begin to interfere with daily life.

Why the Distinction Matters

In food allergies, anxiety and trauma often overlap and are frequently grouped together and labeled simply as "anxiety." However, understanding the difference is important:

- Anxiety is driven by *what might happen* and often responds well to planning, education, and gradual exposure.

- Trauma is driven by *what has already happened* and may require a more body-based, trauma-informed approach that focuses on safety, regulation, and processing past experiences.

Research indicates that children with food allergies experience elevated rates of clinically significant anxiety, with over one-third meeting clinical thresholds in some samples (Ho et al., 2024). A substantial proportion of parents of children with food allergies report symptoms consistent with post-traumatic stress, highlighting the potential for allergic reactions to be experienced as traumatic events (Roberts et al., 2021). These findings make sense in the context of living with a medical condition that carries real risk. Recognizing whether you are responding to future uncertainty, past experience, or both can help guide what support may be helpful moving forward.

It is important to recognize that people respond to experiences differently. Two individuals can go through the same allergic reaction or medical event, and one may experience it as traumatic while the other does not. In the same way, feeling anxious or having trauma-related responses does not automatically mean that someone meets criteria for a mental health diagnosis. These experiences are influenced by many factors, including past experiences, nervous system sensitivity, and the level of support available at the time. What matters most is not whether your experience "counts," but how it is affecting your sense of safety, your daily life, and your overall well-being.

Research has shown that caregivers of children with food allergies report significantly elevated levels of stress, anxiety, and reduced quality of life (Knibb & Semper, 2013). Additional studies have found symptoms consistent with post-traumatic stress and anxiety in both children and parents following severe allergic reactions, particularly anaphylaxis (Roberts et al., 2021). Even without a clearly defined traumatic event, the chronic vigilance required to manage food allergies can contribute to what is sometimes referred to as chronic or cumulative stress, which can have similar effects on the nervous system over time.

When Trauma Gets Labeled as "Anxiety"
One of the challenges in this space is that trauma often gets minimized or mislabeled. Anxiety tends to be understood as excessive or irrational worry. Trauma responses, on the other hand, are rooted in real experiences where something *did* happen, or very nearly happened.

When trauma is labeled as "just anxiety," it is possible that:

- The intensity of the experience may not be fully validated

- Individuals may feel misunderstood or dismissed

- Interventions may focus only on thought patterns, without addressing nervous system responses

- Patients may feel frustrated when standard anxiety tools do not fully help, leading to isolation or resistance to further medical or social/emotional supports and interventions

If your fear feels intense, persistent, or out of proportion to your current level of safety, it does not mean you are overreacting. It may mean your nervous system is still responding to something it experienced as threatening.

What Trauma Can Look Like in Food Allergy Life
Trauma responses do not always look dramatic. More often, they are subtle, internal, and easy to overlook. They can show up as intrusive thoughts or vivid memories of past reactions, a heightened sense of vigilance, or a constant scanning for potential risk. Some individuals notice strong physical responses to cues tied to the past, such as certain foods, environments, or even smells. Many also begin avoiding situations that feel threatening despite being medically safe. It can also become difficult to trust safety,

even after appropriate precautions have been taken, and emotional reactions may feel more intense or harder to regulate. Sleep disruption, irritability, and a persistent sense of being "on edge" are also common.

For parents, these responses may take the form of difficulty trusting others to care for their child, ongoing fear even in controlled or familiar environments, and a deep sense of responsibility to anticipate and prevent every possible risk. For children, trauma can present differently, often through resistance to eating, clinginess or distress in any setting but especially those that are food-related, or behavioral changes that reflect underlying fear that may be interpreted as defiance or another behavioral issue.

When the Body Sounds the Alarm
Understanding anxiety and trauma is especially important when considering or beginning immunotherapy. Many patients and families are too afraid to consider food allergy treatment, or have had difficulty moving forward with it due to unaddressed anxiety and trauma that negatively impacts treatment.

When anxiety or trauma responses are activated, they can have a strong influence on how decisions are made about treatment. Families may delay starting a therapy that could be helpful, stop a process prematurely, or make choices based primarily on fear rather than on a balanced understanding of risk and benefit. Patients may resist or avoid participation in ways that are often misunderstood as noncompliance, but are actually rooted in a nervous system trying to stay safe.

The goal is not to eliminate these feelings or to push through them forcefully. Anxiety and trauma responses carry important information, and they deserve to be acknowledged and felt. At the same time, we want to gently shift toward a place where these feelings are not the sole drivers of our decisions. Instead, we can learn to hold both, honoring the emotional experience while still making thoughtful, values-based choices about treatment and care.

Anxiety, Trauma, and Treatment
Many patients and parents pursue treatment with thoughtful, well-informed intentions, pushing through initial resistance in hopes that the up-front stress of treatment will lead to improvement overall once maintenance is reached. Quality of life does usually improve following treatment for patients (Anagnostou et al., 2014) and parents (Arasi et al., 2014), but anxiety may become a barrier to completing therapy and is the reason many discontinue treatment (Trevisonno et al., 2024).

Some patients, both children and adults, become highly anxious about dosing and begin to resist or refuse it. Others develop behavioral or emotional changes that begin to affect their daily life. Some experience such strong physical anxiety symptoms that it becomes difficult to tell the difference between anxiety and an allergic reaction. In some cases, children quietly begin avoiding doses altogether, hiding or discarding them because the experience feels too intense to tolerate. These are not signs that something has gone wrong or that anyone has failed. They are signs that the body's alarm system is highly activated and requires support.

Understanding the Symptom Overlap
The symptoms of anxiety, trauma, and allergic reactions can feel remarkably similar in the body. This overlap can create a confusing and sometimes distressing experience, and is highly relevant to the

immunotherapy process because patients and their caregivers are carefully monitoring for signs of a reaction after dosing.

Below are some of the most common symptoms of an allergic reaction, alongside ways that anxiety can create or mimic similar sensations.

- *Tightness in the throat*
  Anxiety can cause the muscles in the throat to tighten, creating a sensation of constriction or difficulty swallowing. This is a common stress response and does not necessarily mean the airway is closing.

- *Shortness of breath or difficulty breathing*
  When anxious, breathing can become shallow or rapid. This can create the feeling of not getting enough air, even when oxygen levels are normal.

- *Chest tightness*
  The body's stress response can cause muscle tension in the chest, which can feel similar to the pressure and discomfort experienced during an allergic reaction.

- *Coughing*
  Anxiety can trigger throat irritation or a dry cough, especially when someone becomes hyper-aware of their breathing or throat sensations.

- *Stomach discomfort or nausea*
  The digestive system is closely connected to the nervous system. Anxiety can slow digestion or create nausea, cramping, or a "sick" feeling in the stomach.

- *Flushing or warmth*
  Stress can cause changes in blood flow, leading to warmth or redness in the skin.

- *Itching or tingling sensations*
  Heightened awareness of the body, combined with stress, can create or amplify sensations like itching, tingling, or "something feels off."

- *Dizziness or lightheadedness*
  Changes in breathing patterns during anxiety can lead to feeling faint or unsteady.

Each of these symptoms can be a real physical experience, and each can understandably trigger concern in someone who is actively ingesting their allergen and monitoring for signs of an allergic reaction.

The Cycle That Can Develop

When these sensations occur, especially during or after dosing, the mind naturally tries to interpret them. When one is uncertain whether these are an allergic reaction, of course anxiety increases. As anxiety increases, the body produces more physical symptoms. Those symptoms then reinforce the fear that something is wrong. This can create a cycle that is easily triggered and difficult to break.

What Treatment Asks of Us

Immunotherapy treatment asks the nervous system to do something very specific and difficult. It asks you or your child to move *toward* something that has previously been associated with danger, that you have been carefully moving *away* from to stay safe. Even in a medically supervised setting, this can activate deeply learned protective responses. It is extremely important to get clear guidance from your allergist before beginning treatment. Knowing exactly what to look for, when to act, and what to do can help reduce uncertainty and support more confident decision-making.

If anxiety or trauma are present and unaddressed, starting treatment can feel overwhelming or unmanageable. If anxiety or trauma existed prior to considering treatment and is still significantly impacting daily life, it is often helpful to address that first with the support of a mental health professional. If trauma develops during treatment, possibly after a reaction or difficult experience, it may be important to pause, slow down, or adjust the process while that experience is processed and integrated. This does not mean treatment has failed. It means the nervous system needs support.

What This Book Can and Cannot Do

This book can help you recognize when your experience may involve trauma and normalize and validate those responses. It provides tools to support regulation and reflection to help you make informed, emotionally aware decisions. The activities may help you address stress and anxiety that arise in the course of decision-making and treatment. However, this book cannot give you a comprehensive understanding of anxiety or trauma and related mental health diagnoses.

If you recognize yourself or your child in this section and the activities shared here are not helpful in addressing your concerns, support from a licensed mental health professional with training and experience in trauma work is strongly recommended. The following activities are designed to help you determine whether you could benefit from that type of support, not for diagnostic purposes.

Is This Trauma?: Understanding Your Experience

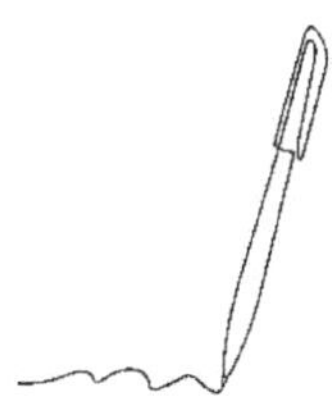

This worksheet is designed to help you reflect on whether your or your child's experience
may include trauma-related responses, and whether additional support may be helpful.

Past Experiences

Have you/your child experienced any of the following?

☐ Severe allergic reaction (anaphylaxis)　　☐ Emergency room visit related to allergies

☐ Reaction that felt unexpected or confusing　　☐ A close call or near exposure

☐ Ongoing fear related to unpredictability　　☐ Epinephrine use

Notes:

____

____

Current Responses

In the present, do you notice any of the following?

☐ Strong fear or distress in food-related situations

☐ Difficulty trusting safety even when reassured

☐ Avoidance of foods or situations that are medically safe

☐ Physical symptoms (racing heart, tight chest, nausea) when thinking about/encountering allergens

☐ Intrusive thoughts or memories about past reactions

☐ Memories or dreams about a past experience

☐ Feeling constantly "on alert"

Notes:

____

____

What areas of daily life are impacted?

☐ Eating　　　　　　☐ Social activities　　　　　☐ School or work

☐ Emotional wellbeing　　☐ Relationships　　　　　☐ Energy levels

☐ Physical wellbeing (pain, tension)　☐ Memory/concentration　　☐ Sleep

Notes:

____

____

Reflection

Does this feel more like:

☐ Occasional anxiety that feels manageable

☐ Persistent or intense fear that feels hard to control

☐ Something that feels connected to past experiences

Notes:

____

____

Support Check

Would additional support be helpful right now?

☐ I feel supported and able to manage this

☐ I would benefit from learning more coping strategies

☐ I would like to explore support with a mental health professional

Notes:

____

____

If Starting or Continuing Treatment

Do these responses feel manageable within a treatment setting?
Would it feel helpful to pause, slow down, or prepare more emotionally first?

Notes:

____

____

Closing Reflection

"A nervous system responding in these ways makes sense based on what it has experienced. Support is available, and I do not have to navigate this alone."

Trauma, Coping Patterns, and the Nervous System in Food Allergy Families

 Many food-allergic adults seeking therapy report that they are "just an anxious person." Parents often describe their food-allergic children's behaviors as personality rather than responses to stress. When we look closely at these patterns through the lens of trauma, we can see that what feels like personality can also be the nervous system's way of keeping us safe.

Trauma is not only something that happens in dramatic, life threatening events. Trauma can arise from *perceived* threat or danger, not just from the actual severity of the event as it occurred. This means that someone can have a trauma response even without experiencing a severe reaction. The nervous system can register events as dangerous even when there was no physical harm. Those who have experienced or witnessed their child experience health emergencies often describe a moment when they felt powerless, terrified, frozen, or consumed by fear. These moments can shape the nervous system in ways that remain active long after the event itself.

Trauma affects the nervous system and the brain in specific ways. It increases alertness to potential danger, amplifies physical sensations of threat, and creates patterns of avoidance or hypervigilance. Over time these patterns become familiar, automatic ways of responding (Teicher & Samson, 2016). This helps explain why someone may feel fine in everyday situations but experience intense stress around health news, allergy conversations, or medical procedures.

You do not have to consciously remember every moment of trauma to be impacted by it. Memories formed before verbal language can still shape the nervous system. Research shows that preverbal experiences are stored differently in the brain but still influence behavior and physiological response later in life (Gentsch & Kuehn, 2022). In the context of food allergies, a child's first reaction or medical encounter might have occurred so early that the narrative memory is faint or absent, yet the body still remembers. These early experiences can shape how they respond to food discussions, doses, medical environments, and even subtle reminders.

Trauma can also affect relationships within families. Parents who fear for their child's safety can become hypervigilant, which children can feel as pressure or anxiety (Afzal et al., 2022). Children who have repeated stress around allergies can become avoidant or shut down. These patterns are not simply personality traits. They are adaptations to the environment in which the nervous system learned to keep the person safe.

The following worksheet helps you reflect on how your own symptoms related to food allergy stress and trauma show up.

Visual Body Map

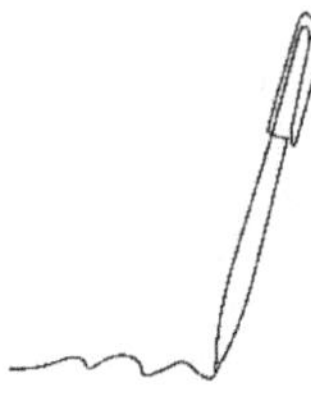

Choose a body map from the following pages to help you notice where you experience physical sensations during moments of allergy-related stress or uncertainty. You may use words, symbols, or colors. There are no right or wrong answers.

On the body map:

Mark areas where you notice sensations during anxiety.

Use a different color or mark for sensations you have experienced during allergic reactions.

Circle areas where you experience overlap of both allergy and anxiety symptoms.

Reflection questions:

Which areas of my body tend to have the fastest or strongest reactions?

____
____
____

Are there sensations that show up both during anxiety and during allergic reactions?

____
____
____

How do I differentiate between anxiety and an allergic reaction in those areas?

____
____
____

Which sensations tend to escalate my worry the fastest?

____
____
____

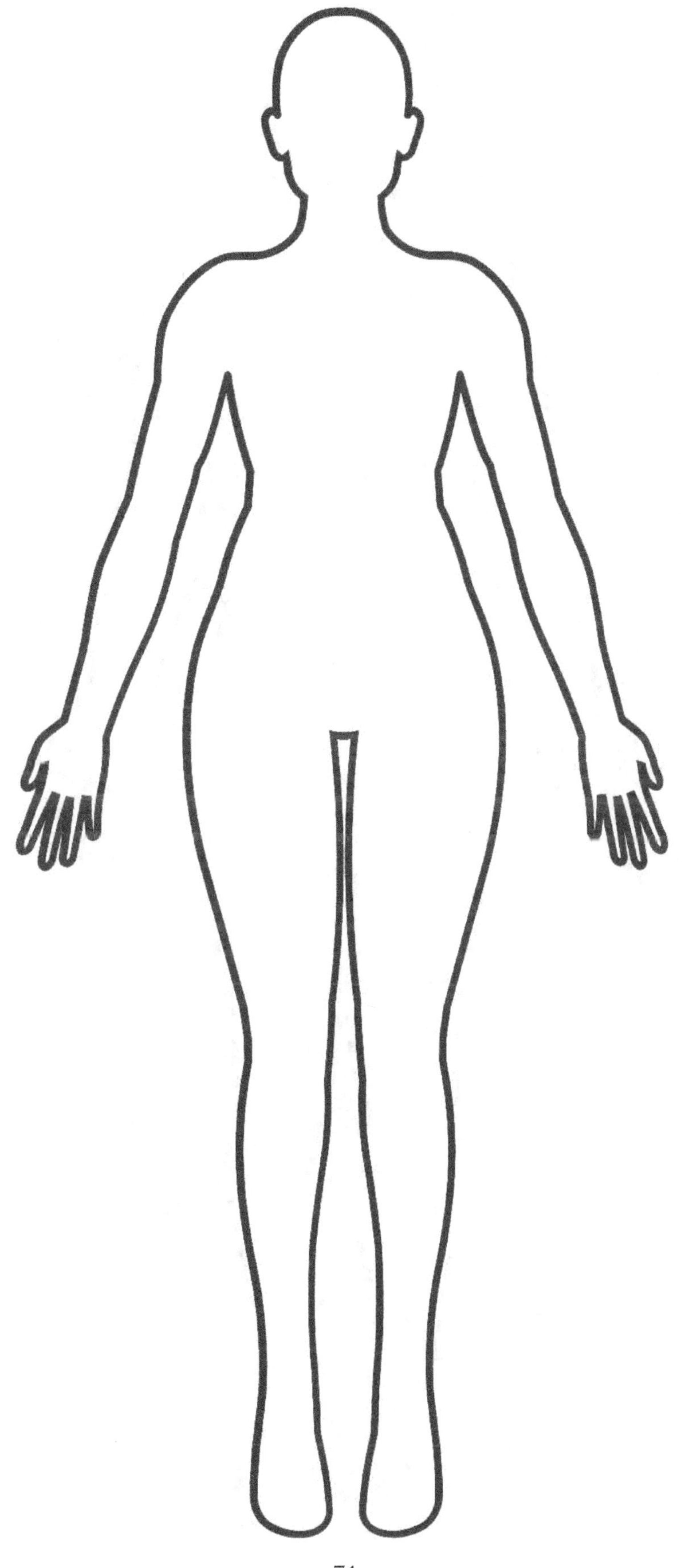

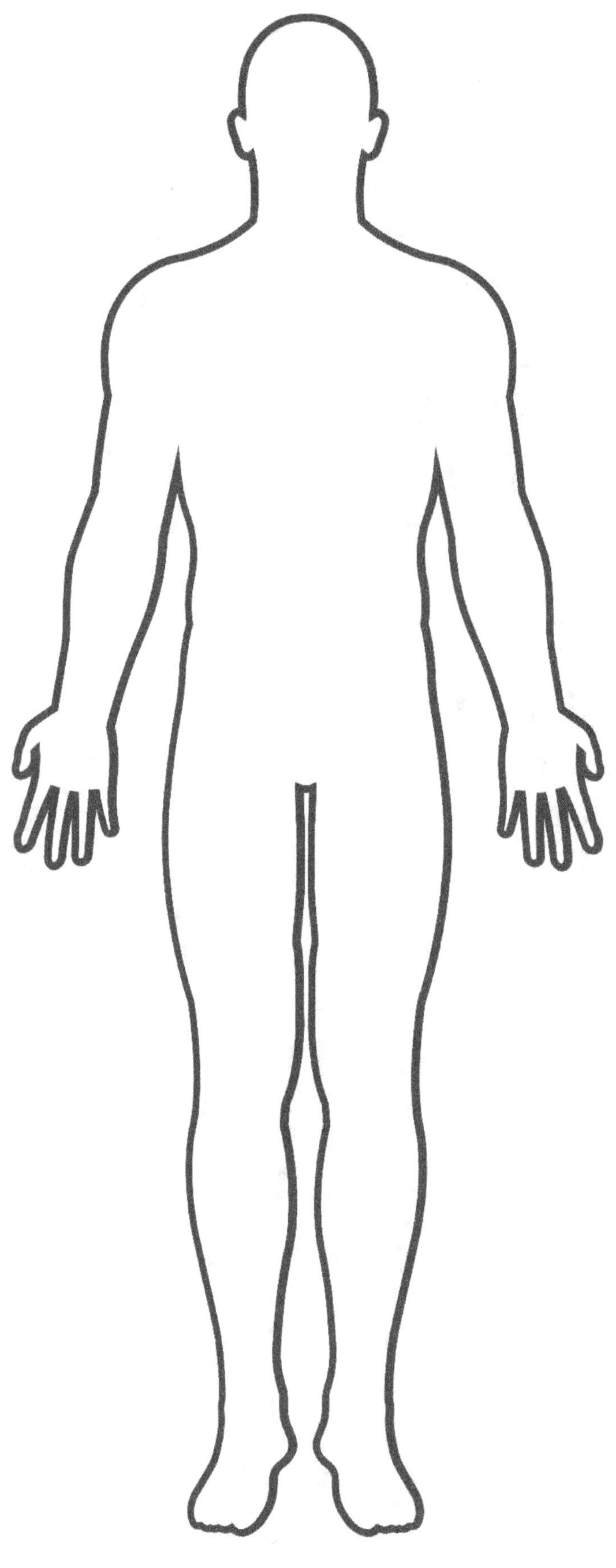

Exploring Symptoms Together

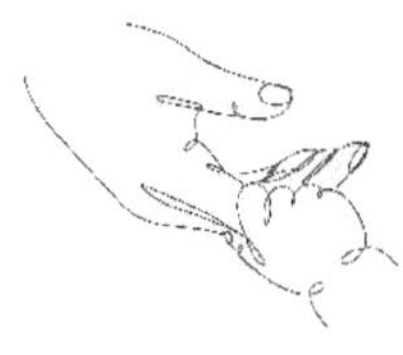

Materials Needed: Two colors of sticky notes (or two colors of stickers)

Instructions for the Adult

This activity helps your child see the difference between physical signs of an allergic reaction and physical signs of anxiety. The focus is on understanding, not dismissing feelings.

List Common Symptoms Together

Sit with your child and a calm voice say:

"Some feelings in our bodies come from allergies. Some come from worry. Let's talk about them together so we can understand them better."

Allow your child to speak first and identify symptoms of an allergic reaction or worry that they can remember. Then prompt them gently with experiences they have had. You don't need to cover all these symptoms, just those they have experienced.

- *Skin:* rash, itchy, bumps, pale
- *Breathing:* heavy breathing or tight chest, coughing, wheezing
- *Stomach:* belly ache, tummy feels funny, throwing up, diarrhea
- *Heart:* heart beats fast
- *Head:* woozy or light
- *Mouth and tongue:* itchy, thick, swollen
- *Eyes:* puffy, itchy, watery, teary, red
- *Nose:* sneezy, runny, stuffy, itchy
- *Voice:* hoarse, hard to speak, tight

Post-it Mapping

- As each symptom is named, ask your child where they feel it on their body.
- Place a sticky note for allergy-related symptoms on the body part that matches the symptom.
- Place a sticky note of another color for worry-related symptoms on the body..
- Place the sticky notes on the child's body/clothing for a more playful exercise. If they prefer, allow them to choose a body map from the pages that follow.

Follow your child's lead by repeating their language and expanding on it

- "Where do you feel itchy skin?"
- "When your tummy feels funny from worry, where do you feel it?"
- "Does your heart beat fast when you are scared or when you are worried about food?"

Notice Overlap

Once all notes are placed, say:
"Let us look together at where the colors are. See how some of these feelings happen in the same places? That is why it can be hard to tell what is happening, even for adults."

Validate

"Both kinds of feelings are real. One tells us about our body's safety and one tells us about our worry. It is okay to have both."

Closing Reflection

Explore what you noticed together. Some questions you might ask include:

- "What parts of your body did we notice feelings in?"
- "What places did we see both colors and why?"
- "How does it feel to learn about these together?"

Validate their experience. Reassure them that understanding sensations helps them feel safer and more confident.

Please note: This worksheet is intended to help you better understand the overlap between anxiety and allergy symptoms, but it is not a tool for diagnosing or determining when to treat an allergic reaction. Always follow your individualized allergy action plan as developed with your physician. If you are ever unsure whether symptoms may be related to an allergic reaction, treat according to your allergy action plan and seek medical guidance immediately. Be sure to review any questions or uncertainties about symptoms and treatment decisions with your healthcare provider.

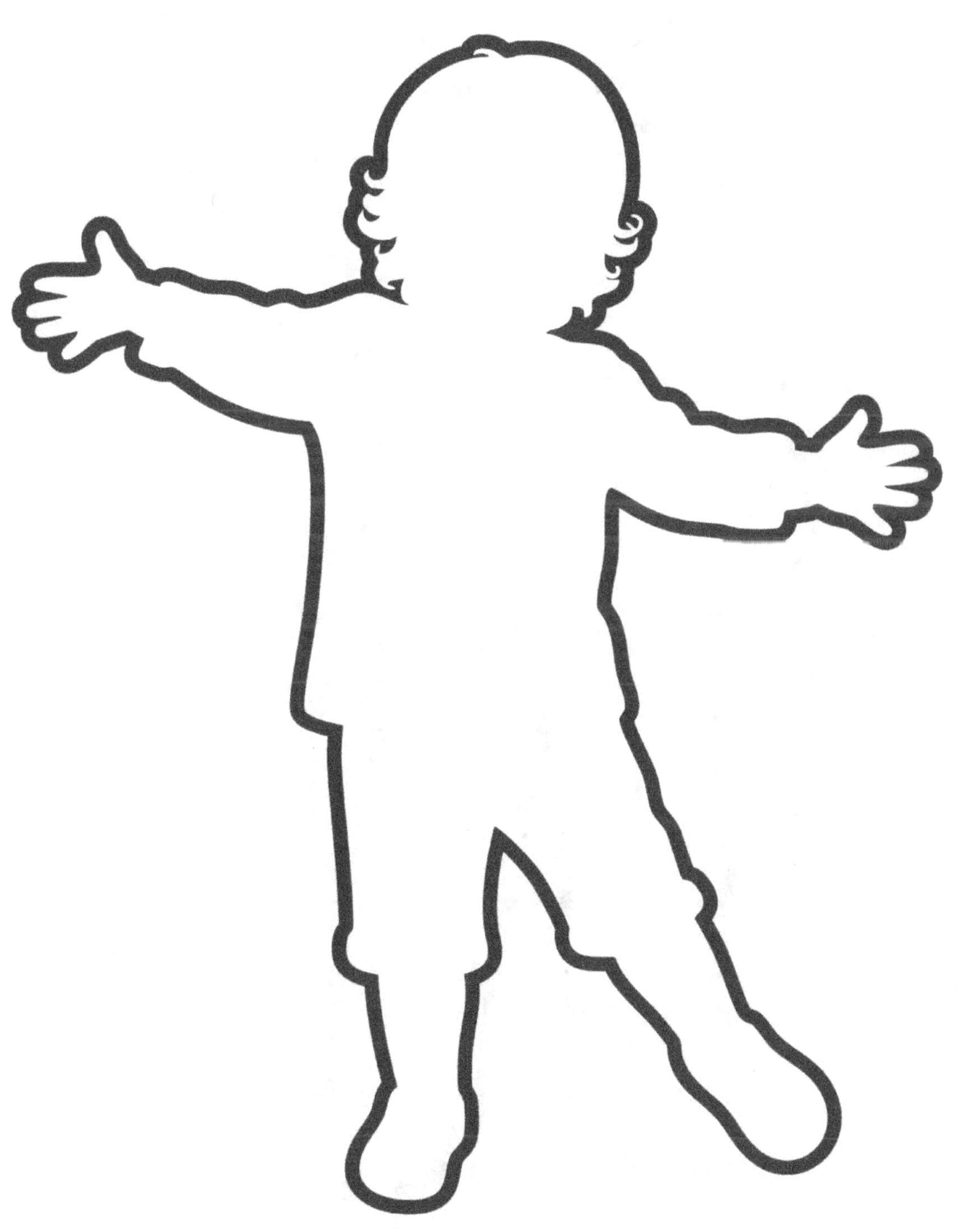

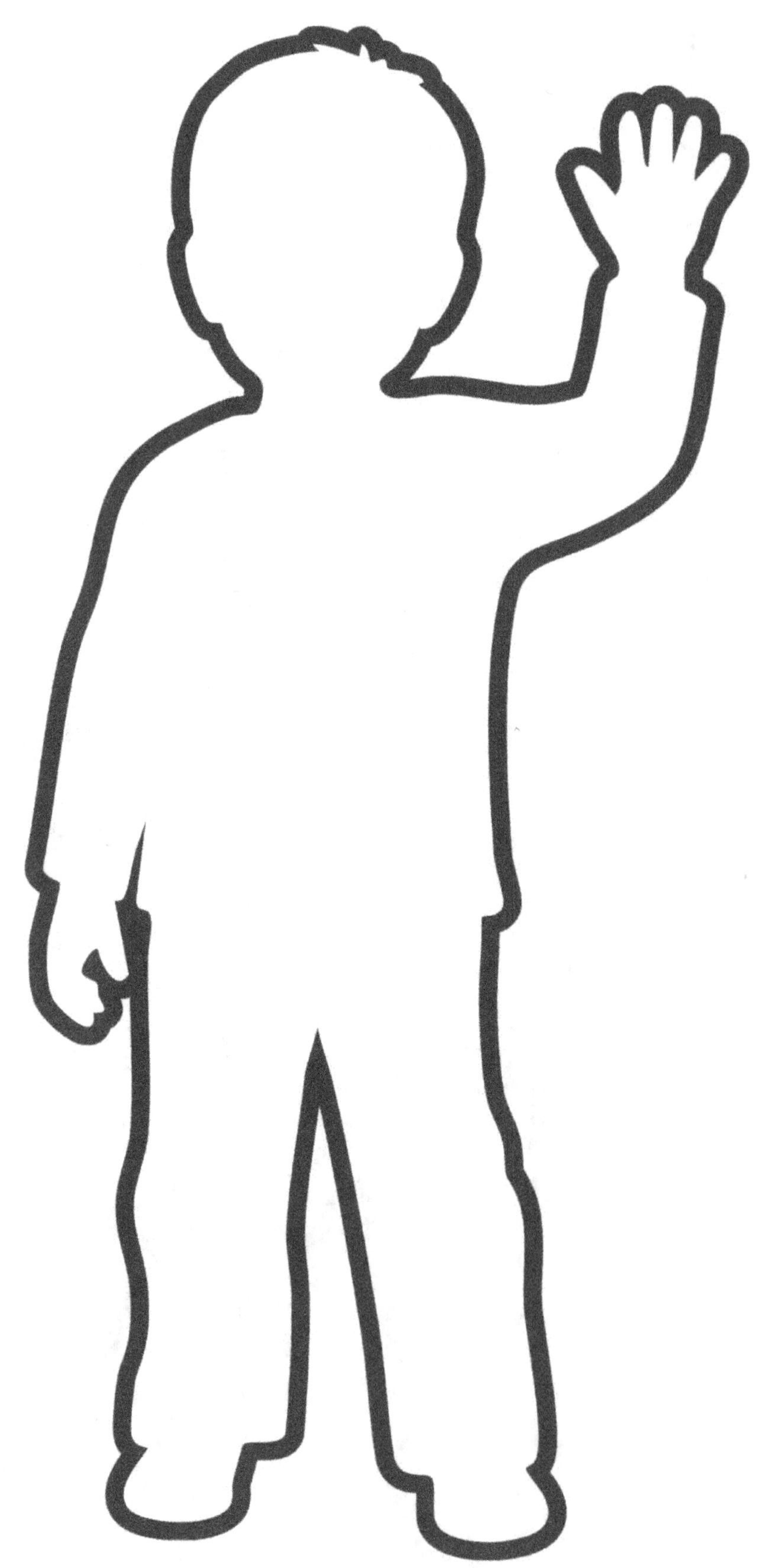

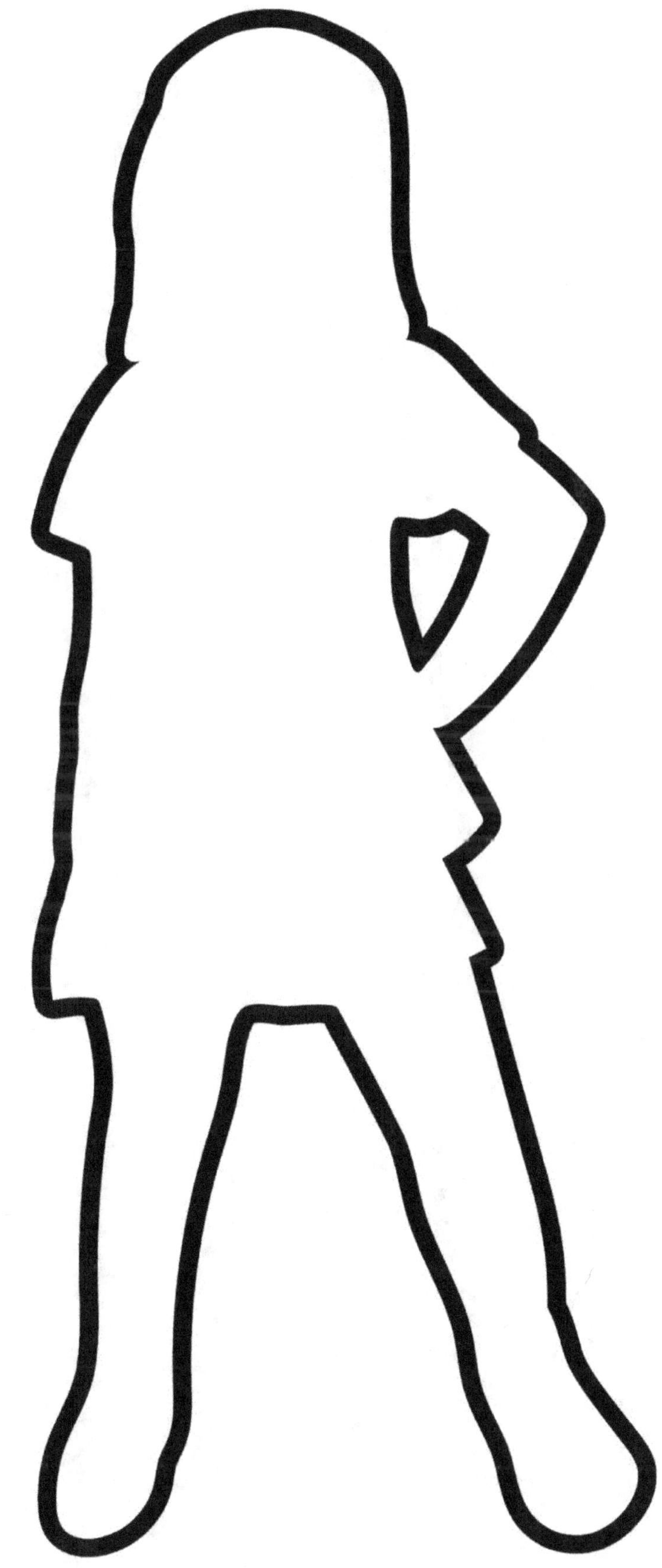

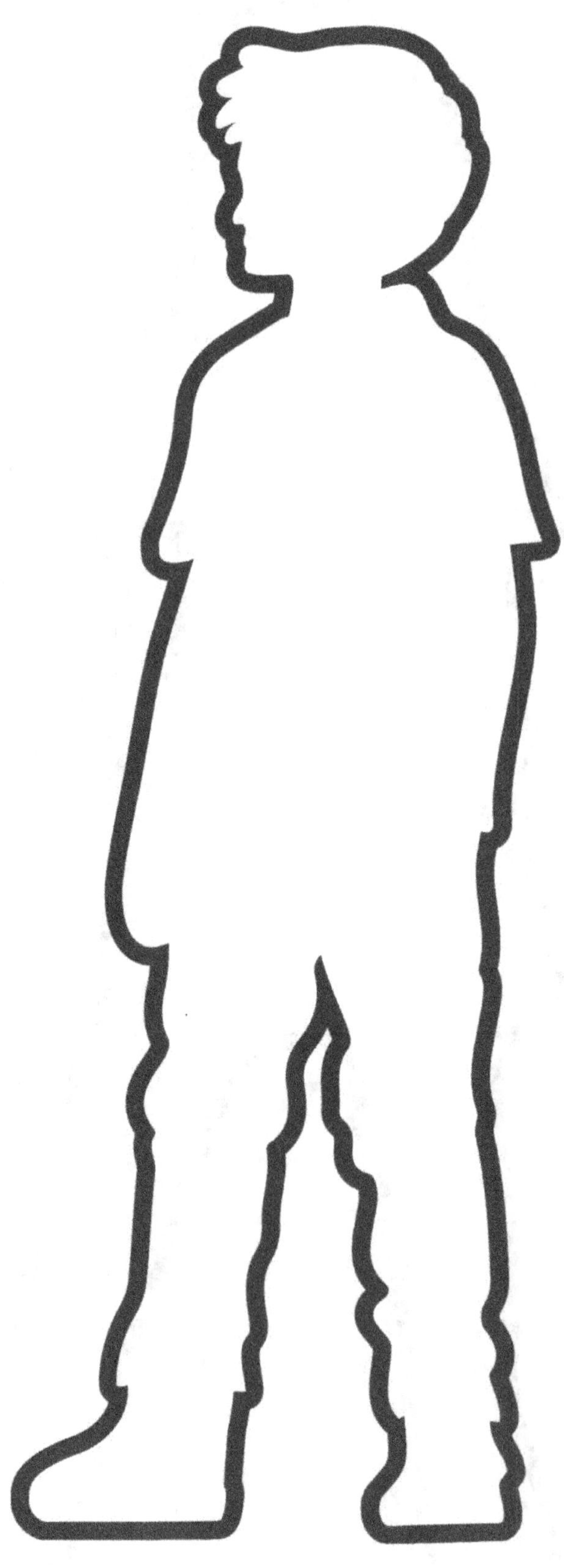

Communication as a Foundation for Treatment Success

 Each day of our lives is filled with moments where we communicate, usually without thinking about it. If we pause and pay closer attention, we might notice that the way we speak shifts depending on the context or who we are with. In moments of stress or urgency, it is easy to move quickly into problem-solving, reassuring, or directing others toward what we think they should feel or do.

Phrases like "don't be scared," "you're fine," or "it's okay" are common and usually offered with good intentions. They are meant to comfort, to move things along, or to reduce distress. But they can unintentionally send the message that an emotion is too much, inconvenient, or not quite right.

This matters in every relationship, but it becomes especially important when we are supporting children. The way we communicate with them helps shape how they understand their own internal experiences. It teaches them whether their feelings are safe to express, whether they will be heard, and how to make sense of what is happening in their bodies and minds.

In the context of medical care, and especially immunotherapy, communication carries even more weight. Success is not only about following a protocol. It is also about creating an ongoing dialogue that makes space for the child's experience, supports regulation, and builds trust over time. How we speak, respond, and listen in these moments becomes part of the treatment itself.

Listening: The Heart of Good Communication

Good communication begins with listening. When under stress, it is natural to offer advice, reassurance, or solutions. We want to fix the problem quickly, eliminate the anxiety, or protect others from feeling upset. Yet the most important first step in any meaningful conversation is simply to pause and listen.

Listening is more than hearing words. It is noticing tone, body language, facial expressions, and energy. It is giving full attention to the other person, even when what they are saying is uncomfortable or difficult or something we may already know but they need to express. Children are especially sensitive to both what we say and how we say it. Our posture, gestures, tone of voice, and even small facial expressions communicate as much as words. When we are rushed, stressed, or anxious, our nervous systems can influence our communication, sometimes making our words come across as harsh, hurried, or critical.

What Good Listening Looks Like

Good listening is active and attuned, allowing the speaker to feel heard and understood. Some key aspects include:

- *Eye contact:* Appropriate to others' comfort, signaling presence without pressure
- *Body language:* Open, calm posture; uncrossed arms; relaxed shoulders
- *Tone of voice:* Steady, gentle, and patient; avoiding sharpness or rushing
- *Verbal encouragement:* Simple acknowledgments like "I hear you," "Thank you for telling me"
- *Reflection:* Restating what you heard in your own words to confirm understanding

- *Patience:* Allowing pauses and giving space for the speaker to continue without interrupting or immediately problem-solving

What ineffective listening looks like:

- Interrupting, rushing, or finishing sentences for someone else
- Offering reassurance before the person has fully expressed themself
- Telling the speaker how they "should" feel
- Displaying visible tension, distraction, or impatience
- Disinterest or empty replies ("uh huh")

The Power of Questions

Open-ended questions invite reflection, dialogue, and understanding. They cannot be answered with a simple yes or no. These questions encourage the speaker to explore and describe their feelings, thoughts, and experiences, and allow the listener to gain insight into their perspective.

Examples of open-ended questions include:

- "What part of this feels toughest for you?"
- "How did that experience make you feel?"
- "Can you tell me more about what you noticed?"

Reframing questions is another useful strategy. Reframing shifts the focus from judgment, assumptions, or reassurance to curiosity and understanding. For example:

- Instead of asking, "Are you scared?" try "What about this feels scary?"
- Instead of "Are you okay?" ask "How are you feeling right now?"
- Instead of "Are you ready to dose now?" try "What would make this easier for you to try?"

Why Listening and Helpful Questions Matter

Children often receive messages about their feelings and experiences through tone and response, not just words. When adults truly listen and respond with curiosity, children feel safe naming and exploring their emotions. This is especially important during medical treatments like immunotherapy, where anxiety, fear, and uncertainty are natural. By listening first and asking thoughtful questions, we help children process emotions, regulate their nervous system, and feel more confident navigating challenging experiences.

Why It Is So Hard to Validate Our Children's Difficult Feelings

As parents, most of us want to protect our children from discomfort. When a child experiences fear, frustration, anxiety, or sadness, especially around something as emotionally charged as a medical procedure or food allergy management, our instinct is often to step in, fix the problem, or reassure them that everything will be okay. We often speak for them in medical settings in the interest of accuracy. We might also be conscientious of our medical providers' time and rush them to stay on schedule. There are many reasons we could rush children through a difficult feeling or try to minimize it, even when our intentions are loving and supportive.

Another difficult aspect of this is that our children's intense emotions can trigger our own. Watching a child feel scared or overwhelmed can stir up our own anxiety, memories of past difficulties, or feelings of helplessness. In those moments, it is natural to want to take control, soothe, or distract, but this can inadvertently teach children that their emotions are too big to be handled safely.

Many parents fear that acknowledging a child's distress will amplify it. We worry that by naming the fear or sadness we will make it worse, as if drawing attention to it somehow gives it power. We also fear feeling helpless ourselves because we cannot instantly make the distress disappear. In a world that often values productivity and problem-solving, sitting with a child in discomfort can feel uncomfortable, inefficient, or even wrong.

Cultural messages may also encourage us to suppress or "fix" emotions rather than explore them. Parents may have been raised with similar approaches and may not have experienced safe modeling for handling intense emotions. In moments of stress, the nervous system narrows our focus: we become solution-oriented, tense, or reactive, which can unintentionally communicate to the child that their feelings are unsafe, unwelcome, or overwhelming.

Why Validation Works

Research in child development and emotion regulation shows that labeling and validating children's emotions decreases their intensity (Lieberman et al., 2007). When a child feels that their emotions are recognized and accepted, the nervous system interprets the situation as safe and manageable. Validation helps the child move from a state of heightened arousal to a calmer, more regulated state.

Validation can take many forms:

- *Naming and reflecting:* "I see that you feel really nervous about today's dose. That makes sense, This is a big step."
- *Acknowledging legitimacy:* "It's normal to feel scared when something is new and uncertain."
- *Safe presence:* Sitting together calmly, making eye contact, and offering gentle reassurance that they are not alone.

Evidence from developmental psychology and attachment research supports this approach. For instance, studies on emotion coaching show that children whose caregivers validate and help them label emotions demonstrate stronger emotional regulation skills, less intense and shorter-lived negative emotions, and greater resilience in the face of stress (Gottman, Katz, & Hooven, 1997). Validation is not permissive; it does not mean allowing unsafe behavior or letting children avoid responsibility. It simply communicates that emotions themselves are manageable and acceptable.

Part of the power of validation comes from co-regulation, which is when someone feels supported in managing their emotional and physiological responses through connection, presence, and attuned communication. Co-regulation is a powerful safety signal to the nervous system. In the context of food allergies and other medical needs, this becomes especially important. Children look to their parents not only for information about safety, but also for cues about how to feel in response to a situation. A calm, steady, and responsive caregiver can help a child's nervous system settle, even during stressful experiences like reactions, medical procedures, or treatment dosing. Over time, these repeated experiences of co-regulation help children build their own capacity for self-regulation. This means that how we communicate can directly influence how our children experience and cope with their medical care (Feldman, 2007).

How to Validate Without Amplifying Fear

Parents often worry that acknowledging emotions will intensify them. The key is to validate in a calm, grounded way without adding extra words of caution or judgment that might escalate anxiety. Some important things to practice are:

- *Stay calm yourself:* Your tone of voice, breathing, and posture set the stage for the child's nervous system to follow.
- *Name, don't dramatize:* Label the emotion simply without exaggerating the situation.
- *Reflect without fixing:* Show that you understand the feeling without immediately offering solutions or reassurance.
- *Avoid minimization or dismissal:* Phrases like "Don't worry" or "It's not a big deal" often make children feel unheard and can amplify their sense of danger.
- *Focus on presence over problem-solving:* Sometimes, simply being there and listening fully is more helpful than any advice.

For example, instead of saying, "Don't be afraid of the shot, it's fine," you could say, "I see this shot feels scary to you. That makes sense and it's okay to feel that way. I'll be right here with you."

When validation is practiced consistently, children learn that their feelings can be acknowledged and tolerated. They internalize the message that emotions, even big or uncomfortable ones, are safe to experience. Over time, this not only reduces the intensity of distress but also strengthens the parent-child relationship, builds trust, and supports the child in navigating challenges independently.

Using "I'm Noticing" to Build Awareness

One of the simplest ways to support your child's emotional awareness without adding pressure or judgment is to start with the phrase, *"I'm noticing…"*

This small shift in language changes the tone of the interaction. Instead of correcting, labeling, or assuming, you are gently reflecting what you observe. It keeps the focus on curiosity rather than criticism, and it gives your child space to recognize their own internal experience.

For example, instead of asking your child why they are upset, or telling them to calm down, you could say, "I noticed that you got quiet after we left for your appointment," or "I am noticing that your body looks tense right now." These statements do not tell your child what they *should* feel. They simply bring attention to what is already happening.

From there, you can gently invite them to share more with open-ended questions like, "Can you tell me how you're feeling?" Even if your child doesn't respond right away, you are helping them build an important skill: noticing their own thoughts, feelings, and body signals. Over time, this kind of language supports emotional awareness, regulation, and trust.

You don't need to get it exactly right. The goal is not to interpret and label things perfectly, but to stay curious, open, and connected as you help your child make sense of their experience.

Nonverbal Communication

Good communication is not only what we say; it is also how we say it and what our bodies convey. Children are highly attuned to stress cues in parents. A hurried tone, sharp instructions, or tense posture can communicate worry, urgency, or frustration even when the words themselves are neutral. A calm, steady voice, open posture, and slow pace can signal safety and presence, even in a stressful moment.

This is particularly relevant in immunotherapy or other medical experiences that are emotionally charged. You may feel nervous, uncertain, or worried, and those emotions will naturally come through. Awareness of your own nonverbal cues allows you to model regulation and provide reassurance, while still acknowledging that it is okay to feel stressed. Remember, the goals are attunement and presence.

Ongoing Dialogue

Good communication with your child in the context of allergy treatment looks like:

- *Involving your child in decision-making, to an age-appropriate degree.*
  Even young children benefit from knowing they have a voice, whether it is choosing the snacks, order of necessary steps in a routine, or naming their feelings in their own words. Older children and teens can be partners in more complex conversations about treatment goals, expectations, and potential challenges.
- *Explaining the process clearly, using words and examples that match their developmental level.*
  Check for understanding rather than assuming comprehension. Encourage questions and curiosity.
- *Ongoing conversation about progress, challenges, and experiences.*
  Ask open-ended questions like, "How did that dose feel?" or "What did you notice today?" and truly listen without inserting assumptions or immediate corrections. This helps you learn what is working, what is stressful, and where additional support is needed.
- *Validating their physical and emotional experiences.*
  When a child reports symptoms or discomfort, it is important to hear them fully without overemphasizing or minimizing. "I'm sorry that your stomach feels funny. We'll keep an eye on it together" communicates acknowledgment without unnecessary alarm.

While this workbook cannot provide a comprehensive guide to communication, the principles above can serve as a foundation: slow down, notice your patterns, pay attention to what your body is communicating, and prioritize listening and understanding over fixing or directing. Over time, these practices help children feel safe, heard, and capable, qualities that support emotional well-being, a strong parent-child relationship, and the success of medical treatments like immunotherapy.

Resources for learning more about communication:

- Daniel Siegel: *The Whole-Brain Child* and *Parenting from the Inside Out*
- Adele Faber and Elaine Mazlish: *How to Talk So Kids Will Listen and Listen So Kids Will Talk*
- Brene Brown: *The Gifts of Imperfection* and *Atlas of the Heart* (for parent reflection)

Nonverbal Communication

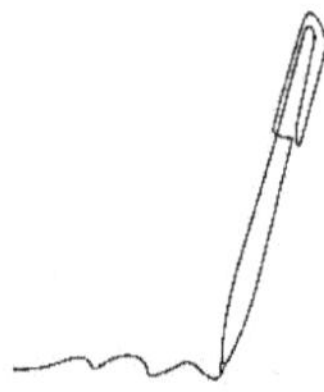

What am I really saying? Over the course of a few days, use this chart to observe and reflect on your own nonverbal signals toward your child. Notice how often they match or contradict what you want to communicate.

Use tally marks and/or make notes to help you explore your own patterns.

Nonverbal Cue:	Connecting Actions	Disconnecting Actions
Tone of Voice/ Volume	calm, steady, warm, even, comforting	sharp, rushed, loud, monotone, flat, tense
Facial Expression	gentle smile, soft eyes, relaxed face, neutral expression	furrowed brow, tight jaw, frowning, expressionless, pursed lips
Posture/ Body Orientation	open posture, relaxed shoulders, kneeling/bending to their level	arms crossed, leaning away, hands clenched, hands on hips, hovering over
Gestures/ Hand Movement	slow and open gestures, open palms	pointing, throwing arms up, shaking head
Eye Contact	maintained softly, nodding to show listening	avoiding eyes, staring too intensely, looking around or at floor
Physical Touch	gentle pat, hand on shoulder, high-five, fist bump, holding hands	absent touch, abrupt, tense, forced, pulling away when touched/reached for
Proximity/ Personal Space	comfortable distance, moves closer if invited (based on child's signs)	too close or too far, invading space, stepping back, leaning away
Pauses/ Pace of Speech	pausing to listen, speaking slowly	too fast, cutting off pauses, interrupting
Mirroring/ Matching Energy	matching tone/gestures/body language, repeating child's words back to them	faster/slower than child, overly intense/serious/silly

Reflection:

Which nonverbal cues do I most commonly use that match what I want to communicate?

____

____

____

____

Which cues do I use that might unintentionally contradict my message or create disconnection?

____

____

____

____

How can I adjust my nonverbal communication to feel more attuned with my child or others?

____

____

____

____

Changes I'd like to make based on what I noticed:

____

____

____

____

____

____

The Nervous System and Communication

 Our nervous system plays a central role in whether we can communicate in an attuned way. When we are calm and regulated, our nervous system supports empathy, reflection, and patience. This is why some conversations flow naturally and feel easy, even when they involve complex or emotionally charged topics.

Conversely, when our nervous systems are activated by stress, fatigue, worry, or fear, our communication can be "hijacked." Dysregulation may cause us to:

- Speak sharply or abruptly without intending to
- Interrupt, over-reassure, or offer solutions too quickly
- Minimize or dismiss someone else's feelings
- Overreact to small challenges or perceived slights
- Withdraw, tune out, or become emotionally unavailable

These reactions are the nervous system signaling that it is perceiving threat or overwhelm, not a reflection of our character or parenting. Understanding this connection helps us approach communication with compassion for ourselves as well as others. Recognizing the signs of dysregulation such as racing thoughts, muscle tension, shallow breathing, or emotional reactivity allows us to pause, self-regulate, and re-engage in a way that is attuned rather than reactive.

Attuned Communication: How Connection and Regulation Intersect

Communication is not just about our own words and nonverbal cues. It is also about the way our nervous systems are operating in the moment. Attuned communication happens when we are listening and responding thoughtfully, and noticing how our own emotional and physiological states shape the interaction. It is the difference between simply speaking and truly connecting.

Attuned communication is marked by presence, empathy, and responsiveness. When we are attuned, we can sense so much more than what they are saying including what they are feeling, how their body is responding, and how best to support them in that moment. In a parent-child relationship, this means noticing subtle cues. Noticing a furrowed brow, a hesitation in speech, or a slight change in posture might help us respond in a way that conveys understanding and safety. In interactions with co-parents, partners, medical professionals, or our children, attunement helps create clarity, mutual understanding, and collaboration.

What Attuned Communication Looks Like

Some observable qualities of attuned communication include:

- *Calm and regulated tone:* Our voice conveys steadiness even in stressful situations.
- *Body language that mirrors engagement:* Open posture, eye contact, and gestures that signal attentiveness.
- *Empathy in response:* Recognizing emotions without judgment or immediate problem-solving.
- *Pausing to reflect:* Allowing space for others to speak fully without interruption.

- *Responsiveness over reaction:* Adjusting the conversation based on cues from the other person rather than responding purely from our own assumptions, anxieties, or goals.

Why Attuned Communication Matters

Attuned communication is not a luxury. It is a foundation for trust, learning, and emotional safety. When we communicate in an attuned way, we are supporting the nervous systems of both ourselves and the people we are interacting with. Children feel safer expressing difficult feelings, co-parents and partners feel understood, and medical discussions become more productive. Even brief moments of attunement signal to the body that the environment is safe, which decreases stress and increases the ability to think, plan, and respond rather than react.

Conversely, repeated interactions that are marked by dysregulation or misattunement can increase stress, heighten anxiety, and create cycles of misunderstanding or tension. This is particularly important when managing complex situations like medical treatments or new routines, where anxiety can easily escalate and affect everyone involved.

Coping Patterns and Trauma Responses in the Context of Food Allergy

Before we explore specific emotional reactions and behaviors, it helps to understand the patterns that often shape how people respond to ongoing medical stress. Food allergies are a repeated series of decisions, risks, procedures, and unknowns. Over time, this can influence how both adults and children relate to danger, safety, and care.

Coping styles are the ways we tend to respond when we feel threatened, uncertain, or vulnerable. These patterns are not personality traits or diagnoses. They are adaptive patterns that develop based on lived experience, and they influence our coping lens. Most people do not fit neatly into one category and may move between them depending on the situation.

Moving toward the problem

This style is driven by a strong need for certainty and control. The nervous system looks for safety through vigilance, information-gathering, and action.

In the context of food allergies, this might look like:

- Constantly monitoring symptoms or worrying about hidden exposures
- Repeatedly reviewing test results, food labels, or protocols
- Difficulty tolerating uncertainty between appointments or doses
- Feeling compelled to intervene quickly, even when risk is low
- Increased anxiety before testing, challenges, or new foods
- Strong emotional reactions when others do not take the allergy seriously

This approach can be protective and even lifesaving. It can also be exhausting.

Moving away from the problem

This style prioritizes emotional distance as a way to stay regulated. The nervous system seeks safety by minimizing, delaying, or disengaging.

In the context of food allergies, this might look like:

- Avoiding thinking or talking about allergy risks
- Delaying appointments or avoiding testing
- Hesitation or freeze around epinephrine use or in emergencies
- Downplaying reactions or symptoms
- Feeling overwhelmed by discussions about long-term safety or treatment
- Withdrawing from others after emergencies or hospital visits

This pattern often develops when overwhelm has felt unmanageable in the past. It can help create a calm environment around the allergies, but can lead to missing crucial safety steps.

Balanced and flexible coping
A healthy and balanced coping style allows movement toward or away from a problem depending on what is needed in the moment. The nervous system can tolerate uncertainty while staying responsive.

In allergy-related situations, this might include:

- Following safety protocols without becoming consumed by them
- Trusting medical guidance while still asking questions
- Using epinephrine when needed without excessive hesitation or panic
- Allowing others to help with care when appropriate
- Recovering emotionally after reactions or hospital visits

This does not mean the absence of fear. It means fear does not run the system.

When Coping Isn't Enough
Coping skills are often the first tools we reach for when something feels hard. They help us manage, regulate, and move through moments of stress or uncertainty. In the context of food allergies, many patients and parents become incredibly skilled at coping. You learn how to prepare, how to plan, how to read labels, how to advocate, and how to stay vigilant. You develop routines that create a sense of safety and predictability in a world that can sometimes feel unpredictable.

These strategies are protective, adaptive, and often necessary, but can be problematic over time. There are moments when the reactions feel bigger than the situation in front of you, when the body responds before the mind can catch up, when reassurance does not fully land, or when coping tools only help temporarily. You may notice that certain situations feel overwhelming in a way that is hard to explain, or that your child's reactions seem intense even when they are medically safe.

When this happens, it is worth reflecting on whether there is something deeper your nervous system is responding to. This is where we begin to move beyond coping and into understanding how our past experiences may be impacting us now.

Noticing Nervous System Cues During Medical Appointments

This reflection activity will help you increase awareness of how the body signals safety or threat in clinical spaces. While answering, imagine a recent appointment and answer the questions while noticing any thoughts, emotions, and sensations in your body.

What sensations do you notice first when you think about medical visits? Tightness, heat, numbness, restlessness, calm?

____

____

Where does your body tend to hold tension in these settings?

____

____

What happens to your breathing when the provider speaks?

____

____

Do you notice changes in your voice, posture, or ability to ask or answer questions?

____

____

What cues from the provider, office staff, and the office environment help your body feel more at ease?

____

____

What cues increase your vigilance or defensiveness?

____

____

Your nervous system gathers information long before your mind makes meaning of it. Learning to listen does not mean you always obey it, but it gives you valuable data.

Noticing Your Child's Nervous System Cues During Medical Appointments

Now reflect on the same questions for your child's body signals safety or threat in clinical spaces. Picture your child's response to different medical experiences and appointments.

What responses does your child exhibit or express when you bring up medical visits?

____

____

Where does your child seem to hold tension in their body in these settings?

____

____

What happens to their breathing when the provider speaks?

____

____

Do you notice changes in their voice, posture, or ability to ask or answer questions?

____

____

What cues from the provider, office staff, and the office environment put your child more at ease?

____

____

What cues increase their vigilance or defensiveness?

____

____

Container Exercise for Adults

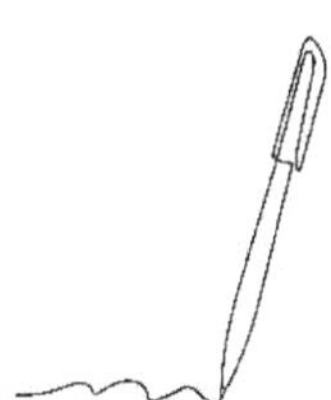

Sometimes difficult emotions need attention, but not in the exact moment they show up. Other times, they can become so big that they overwhelm us, and we need to become more regulated or seek more support before working through them. We often don't have the time, privacy, or nervous system capacity to fully process all our emotions when we feel them.

The container exercise helps us create an intentional pause by visualizing a way to contain big emotions until we are ready to come back to them. This can help reduce overwhelm, increase regulation, and remind your nervous system that you are still in control. This exercise can be used at any time throughout the immunotherapy process or for any other difficult feelings and experiences.

Name What Is Here

What feeling, thought, memory, or fear feels too big right now? (Be as specific as you can.)

Examples:
"I am afraid of the next updose."
"I keep replaying the last reaction."
"I feel angry that this is still so hard."
"I feel guilty about my treatment decision."

Write yours here:

____

____

Create A Container

Imagine a container that feels strong enough and safe enough to hold this for now. It can be anything, and usually the first thing that comes to mind works best. (Examples: a box, a locked drawer, a safe, a suitcase, a jar, a vault, a backpack)

You can also choose to write your emotions down on paper and put them inside an actual physical container.

What does your container look like?

____

____

Why does this container feel safe to you?

____

____

Place the Feeling Inside

Imagine placing the worry, thought, or emotion into the container. As you do, choose a reminder that honors the emotion and your intent.

Examples:
"I am not ignoring this. I will come back to it when I'm ready."
"This matters, and I'll take care of it when I am better able to."
"I can return to this later."

____

____

Choose When You Will Return

Containment works best when your brain trusts that you actually will come back.

When will you revisit this? (Later tonight, after the appointment, once you're home, during therapy, when a trusted friend/partner can be there to support you, in your journal tomorrow)

My time to return to this is:

____

____

Regulate the Present Moment

Now ask what does this moment needs from you right now to regulate and move on to what you need to do next. (Water, food, fresh air, movement, breathing, distraction, support, rest, support)

Right now, I need:

____

____

Final Reflection

Containment is not suppression. It supports regulation and builds self-trust.

It is reminding yourself:

I do not have to process everything at once.
I can feel this and still function.
I can pause without abandoning myself or my emotions.

Container Exercise for Kids

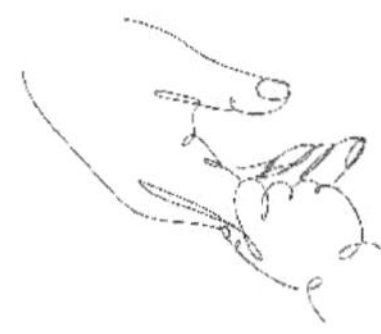 Children often feel big emotions before they have words for them.

Difficult emotions like fear, anger, embarrassment, sadness, and worry usually show up at a time when they can't be fully honored and processed.

The goal is not to make the feelings disappear. It is to help your child learn that feelings are real and important, and we can learn ways to handle them without letting them take over.

A container exercise helps children pause without feeling like they are being told to "stop feeling."

It teaches emotional safety, not emotional avoidance.

Notice Together

Acknowledge the child's emotion without labeling it:
I'm noticing something feels big right now. It seems like this is a hard moment. Is there a big feeling here?

Encourage the child to label the feeling, and give suggestions if they struggle to find words:

Scared / Angry / Sad / Embarrassed / Frustrated / Overwhelmed / Other ______________

What happened right before this feeling showed up?

____

____

Create Their Container

Ask: *If we could put this big feeling somewhere safe for now, what would it go in?*

Let them choose. Make suggestions if they seem stuck: A treasure chest, a superhero vault, a backpack, a dragon cave, a cloud, a jar, a rocket ship, a locked box.

Their answer does not need to make sense to you. It needs to feel safe to them.

Help your child visualize their container by asking questions:

What color is it? How big is it? What does it feel like? Does it have a lock, zipper, lid, or secret code?

Where does it stay when you are not using it? Does it make sounds? Does it sparkle? Is it magical?

Let your child describe it in their own words.

____

____

____

Help Them Place the Feeling Inside

Feelings are important. We can keep them safe until we are ready.

Help them imagine or act out putting their emotions in the container they chose.

Make a Return Plan

Help your child know the feeling will not be forgotten by choosing a time to revisit it?

When should we come back to this?
After school? At bedtime? After the appointment? In the car ride home?

____

____

Help Their Body Feel Safe Now

Ask: *What would help your body move on right now?*

A hug? A drink of water? A walk? Holding your hand? Quiet time? Deep breaths? Music?
A comfort item? A snack? Fresh air? Snuggling a pet?

____

____

Would You Like a Real-Life Version?

It often helps kids to have a real object that matches the container they imagine. Once they are regulated and you have time for an activity, offer to find or create it together. Craft materials and decorations can help kids get excited about this. You may also want to choose a fun notepad or colored sticky note for them to write thoughts and feelings and place them inside.

Ask: *Would you like to make, decorate, or choose a real container like this?*

Write or draw ideas for a real-life container here:

Part III:
Choosing a Path

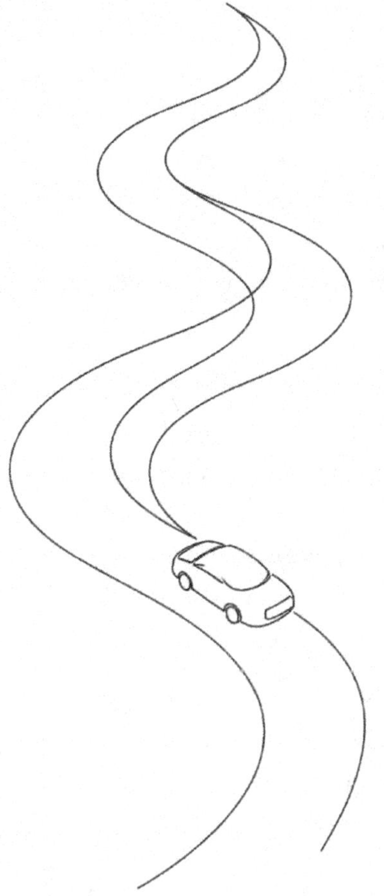

You rarely have time for everything you want in this life,
so you need to make choices. And hopefully your
choices can come from a deep sense of who you are.

— Fred Rogers

Chapter 3:
Shared Decision Making With Your Medical Team

 When navigating treatment options in a rapidly changing landscape, choosing a doctor is the first step in a process of shared decision-making (SDM). Food allergy care has evolved dramatically in the past decade. For many years, the standard message was clear and consistent: strictly avoid the allergen and carry epinephrine.

Up to this point, the decision-making framework has focused on medical variables: diagnosis, reaction threshold, available therapies, comorbid conditions, and measurable risk reduction. These considerations are essential. They create safety. They define options. They establish what is medically possible, but they do not determine what is livable.

A treatment plan can be clinically sound and still feel unsustainable in daily life. A therapy may raise reaction thresholds while simultaneously increasing stress within the family system. A strategy may be medically conservative yet psychologically freeing. Another may be medically proactive but emotionally exhausting. Medical decisions are rarely just medical. They are biopsychosocial decisions. Integrating psychological and lifestyle considerations ensures that treatment adherence is realistic, that anxiety is acknowledged rather than dismissed, and that therapy aligns with long-term functioning rather than short-term intervention.

The next layer of decision-making moves beyond "What works?" to "What works for this person?" Today, families may consider continued avoidance or multiple treatment possibilities, and find themselves having a new kind of conversation with their allergists. Increasingly, doctors are now guiding patients and families through a structured decision-making process grounded in their goals, values, lifestyle, and risk tolerance.

Food allergy management unfolds in kitchens, classrooms, airports, sleepovers, and social gatherings. It lives inside nervous systems that respond to uncertainty with vigilance. It exists within family dynamics, school policies, financial realities, and developmental stages. A toddler's world is different from an adolescent's. A parent with high medical anxiety approaches risk differently than one who feels confident managing reactions. A child with sensory sensitivities may experience daily oral immunotherapy dosing very differently than a peer. There are countless individual factors to consider, making these conversations and decisions quite complex.

Identifying Goals

Dr. Shahzad Mustafa spoke about his approach to these conversations in episode 71 of the *Don't Feed the Fear* podcast (Whitehouse and Mustafa, 2026). Dr. Mustafa is the division head of Allergy, Immunology, and Rheumatology at Rochester Regional Health in Rochester, NY. In addition to seeing both pediatric and adult patients, Dr. Mustafa is involved with teaching medical trainees and participating in clinical research, particularly work on the quality of life considerations in food allergy. Instead of beginning with an explanation of treatment options, Dr. Mustafa first asks patients and families what their goals are. Their answers guide them through a framework for creating a management plan. Here is how Dr. Mustafa shared moving through those discussions:

Step One: Clarify the Goal

Dr. Mustafa begins by asking patients and families what they hope will be different in their lives after allergy treatment. Not every patient wants to eat their allergen regularly. Not every patient wants daily therapy. Some patients and families are comfortable with avoidance, but want protection from accidental exposures. Not every patient is distressed by avoidance and it works well for them. Conversely, not every patient or family feels safe with strict avoidance alone (Whitehouse & Mustafa, 2026).

Goals tend to fall into three broad categories:

1. Maintain avoidance and minimize impact on quality of life.
2. Increase protection against accidental exposure without incorporating the food into the diet.
3. Actively incorporate the allergen into the diet.

Each of these goals leads toward different therapeutic pathways. Without identifying the goal first, families can feel pushed toward interventions that do not actually match their needs.

For example, a teenager allergic to shellfish who has no interest in eating seafood and does not encounter it socially may reasonably choose continued avoidance. In that context, introducing daily therapy may add burden without meaningful benefit. A young child allergic to dairy, wheat or egg who attends daycare and birthday parties often may experience significant quality-of-life limitations that warrant exploring additional protection from accidental exposures, or even consider ways to introduce the food allergen into the diet. The decision-making process must begin with the lived experience of the patient.

Step Two: Confirm the Diagnosis and Understand the Threshold

Before any treatment decision is made, diagnostic clarity is essential. Dr. Mustafa emphasized the role of oral food challenges as the gold standard when appropriate. These are conducted in graded, medically supervised settings and are designed to answer two critical questions: Is the patient truly allergic, and at what dose does a reaction occur?

Thresholds can be important to establish, because a patient who reacts to a trace amount of peanut has a very different risk profile from one who tolerates the equivalent of one or two peanuts before symptoms emerge. Those differences meaningfully influence the decision-making conversation. A higher threshold may offer reassurance with avoidance alone, or allow the patient a higher starting dose and shorter length of immunotherapy treatment. A lower threshold may prompt discussion of protective therapies. Diagnosis and threshold understanding create a foundation built on data rather than assumption (Whitehouse & Mustafa, 2026).

Food challenges are often feared, yet Dr. Mustafa reframed them as both diagnostic and empowering. Research found that when treating anaphylaxis during an in-office food challenge, parents gained confidence in their ability to recognize and treat reactions and reported that the overall experience was positive and helpful (Theodorakakis et al., 2024). Understanding that anaphylaxis is typically responsive to timely epinephrine shifts the narrative from catastrophe to competence.

Step Three: Assess Quality of Life and Daily Burden

Food allergy is a daily lived experience, not just a medical diagnosis. Dr. Mustafa often returns to the concept of quality of life as the primary outcome that matters. Therapies often focus on threshold doses, but the real world aim is to reduce anxiety, emergency visits, and the need for constant vigilance (Whitehouse & Mustafa, 2026).

In clinical conversation, this translates into exploring questions such as:

- How much mental energy is spent managing this allergy each day?
- Does fear of accidental exposure limit social participation?
- Does the allergy cause reluctance to attend events or travel?
- Does the patient/family feel frequent or constant stress?
- How does this patient experience medical procedures?
- What is the patient's/family's tolerance for uncertainty?
- Does daily dosing feel empowering or burdensome?
- Is the anxiety about accidental exposure greater than the anxiety about treatment?

Importantly, interventions can sometimes increase burden rather than relieve it. Daily dosing requirements, frequent office visits, side effects, or the psychological weight of ongoing therapy may not align with a patient or family's capacity or priorities and are some of the most common reasons given for discontinuing OIT (Plessis et al., 2024). Therefore, every intervention must be evaluated through this lens: Can this treatment improve the patient's day-to-day experience?

Step Four: Match the Goal to the Appropriate Strategy

Once goals, diagnostic clarity, and quality-of-life considerations are established, Dr. Mustafa then turns the conversation to aligning therapies with those goals. OIT and SLIT can potentially decrease the immune system's reactivity to a specific allergen long term. The biologic medication omalizumab can provide protection from food allergens, but does not provide long-term effects if the patient stops taking them (Whitehouse & Mustafa, 2026). For those navigating restaurants, travel, and adolescent independence, an additional layer of protection may provide meaningful reassurance.

If the goal includes incorporation of the allergen into the diet, oral immunotherapy may be appropriate, particularly in younger children. Research has shown that OIT is most effective and best tolerated in children ages one to four, with higher rates of successful dietary incorporation in that age group (Vickery et al., 2017). In older children and adolescents, the likelihood of indefinite daily dosing is higher, and adherence becomes an important consideration. Many individual factors shape a careful decision, and no single pathway is universally correct.

Step Five: Evaluate Coexisting Conditions and Systemic Factors

Food allergy rarely exists in isolation. Many patients also have asthma, eczema, allergic rhinitis, or eosinophilic esophagitis, and biologic therapies may offer overlapping benefits. While omalizumab treats asthma and chronic urticaria in addition to food allergy, dupilumab treats eczema, asthma, and eosinophilic esophagitis but has not demonstrated effectiveness for food allergy.

These nuances shape therapy selection. If eczema is the most disruptive condition in a child's life, targeting eczema may take priority over food allergen tolerance. If food-related anxiety dominates daily functioning, treatment may focus there (Whitehouse & Mustafa, 2026). Access to board-certified allergists, insurance coverage, geographic location, and financial realities also influence what is feasible. Shared decision-making must be grounded in these real-world constraints.

Step Six: Reassess Over Time

One of the most important aspects of Dr. Mustafa's approach is recognizing that decisions are not permanent. Food allergy innovation is picking up speed, and what is available to patients will continue changing. Shared decision-making is likely an ongoing conversation that patients and providers will revisit regularly. Continuing to reflect on and adjust treatment decisions is a sign of thoughtful care and learning from valuable experiences, helping you make choices that fit your needs or your child's at different points in your journey (Whitehouse & Mustafa, 2026).

The Heart of the Process

At its core, shared decision-making in food allergy care is not about choosing the most aggressive therapy. It is about choosing the therapy that aligns with the patient's values and improves quality of life. There is no universally right answer, only an answer that fits a person and family in the current season to address their current goals.

The expansion of therapeutic options is an amazing scientific advancement and an invitation to conversation. When that conversation begins with the patient's goal, it shifts the power dynamic from prescription to partnership. In a field that is evolving rapidly, partnership may be the most important innovation of all.

Providers we met along the way

Long before immunotherapy became a plan, I was the Mom with a folder full of research articles tucked under my arm in every appointment. I have always been a reader and a researcher. I am deeply grateful that my formal training in psychology taught me how to find, interpret, and feel confident discussing peer-reviewed scientific information. That ability shaped the very beginning of our journey in ways I could not have anticipated.

In our very first allergist appointment after my son's initial anaphylactic reaction, I listened carefully as the doctor explained how to keep him safe. I was stunned when she gave me factually incorrect or outdated information. These discrepancies made me feel like I had to read and know everything myself because I could not fully trust that our physician would give me accurate information.

Based partly on that interaction, I didn't accept it when she told me with certainty that there was nothing to be done for kids with food allergies other than avoid and prescribe epinephrine. While we settled into the rhythms of strict avoidance, learning labels, cleaning practices, and lifestyle changes, I continued to read and learn. I read about the promising research on oral immunotherapy being conducted at the time, suggesting that controlled gradual exposure to increasing doses of allergens could lead to measurable desensitization and changes in the immune response.

At our next allergy appointment, I arrived not just with questions but with journal articles about research being done on promising innovative treatments. We met with another doctor in the practice who was polite but lukewarm in her response, and before long we received a letter ending our care at that practice. I again felt a wave of discouragement and exhaustion wash over me. It wasn't just that I had to find another doctor. It was that the effort of advocating so fiercely, translating scientific articles into action, and feeling responsible for my son's medical care was exhausting.

I found a new practice where the physicians were willing to coordinate with specialists who understood some of the more nuanced approaches we had been reading about. I remember walking out of that first visit feeling a mix of relief, motivation, cautious hope, and emotional exhaustion. For the first time, my knowledge and engagement were seen as a collaboration rather than a nuisance. My near-constant vigilance shifted slightly and allowed me to exhale. This experience highlighted the importance of shared decision-making, of feeling like you are on the same team as your child's healthcare providers, and of being treated as a valuable partner in care.

After a winding road including both TCM and enrollment in the peanut patch clinical trial, I remained curious about OIT. It hadn't been available near enough to home to make it possible, but I continued to watch and wait hoping someone accessible to us would begin offering it. Eventually, we were incredibly fortunate to connect with a doctor who not only understood my son's high sensitivity and reactivity but also took the time to explain the process, answer my questions, and discuss an individualized approach. He was patient, calm, knowledgeable, and kind. For the first time since I became a parent, I feel seen, taken seriously, and supported as a parent navigating something unfamiliar and emotional.

Meeting him gave me a sense of relief I hadn't expected. For the first time, I felt I could entrust someone else with the weight of my son's care and trust that we were in capable, compassionate hands. Having access to this treatment and a doctor who truly listened made the journey feel possible, and I am deeply grateful for the support and care we received that made it feel possible to take the huge step of beginning OIT.

Choosing a Provider

 Once you've found possible treatment options or paths forward, the next question becomes: who will help guide the journey? In the case of immunotherapy, that role belongs to your allergist. Think of them as the person at the controls: your pilot, your driver, your navigator.

They are responsible for understanding the route, monitoring the conditions along the way, and helping you make adjustments if the path becomes complicated. Choosing a doctor who is experienced, trustworthy, and aligned with your goals can make a significant difference in how the road ahead unfolds.

Provider Qualifications and Experience

Because of this, the first and most important step is making sure the physician guiding you is a board-certified allergist. The field of allergy is expanding rapidly, and staying up-to-date with the changing landscape is extremely important. Food allergy treatment, especially immunotherapy, requires specialized training in the immune system, allergic disease, accurate testing/diagnosis, and the management of allergic reactions. Board certification indicates that the physician has completed rigorous training and maintains updated expertise in allergy and immunology.

The next most obvious factor to consider is which treatments the practice offers. Not every allergist provides the same therapies, and many offer none at all. After learning about the various options available, you may find yourself more interested in one approach than another. Finding a doctor who has experience with the treatment you are considering will be an important part of the decision, and may unfortunately be a barrier to finding the treatment you hope to pursue.

There are also practical realities to consider. Distance from the clinic, frequency of visits, and cost can make a significant difference in day-to-day life. Insurance coverage, out-of-pocket costs, and a clinic's fee structure are also important to understand before starting treatment. Immunotherapy programs vary widely in how they are structured financially, so it is helpful to have a clear picture of what to expect.

Practice Dynamics and Culture

You'll also want to get a feel for the allergist's approach to care and the culture of their practice. Some families value a highly structured program with clear protocols, while others appreciate a practice that emphasizes flexibility and shared decision-making. The way a clinic communicates, educates, and partners with patients and families has a huge impact on the experience.

If you are fortunate enough to have more than one option available to you, it can be helpful to speak with multiple providers before deciding how to proceed. Hearing different perspectives may give you a clearer understanding of your choices. One physician may emphasize a particular treatment approach, while another may recommend a different path based on your medical history and goals. Just as travelers sometimes compare routes before beginning a trip, families can benefit from gathering information before committing to a plan.

It is also important to remember that if your current allergist does not offer a particular treatment or tells you it is not something they provide in their practice, that does not necessarily mean the treatment is inappropriate for you. There are many valid reasons why a physician may choose not to offer a certain therapy. It may reflect the structure of their practice, available resources, or their professional focus, but those practical considerations do not automatically mean that the treatment itself is unsafe or ineffective for a particular patient.

Seeking Additional Opinions

If you are interested in a therapy that your doctor does not provide, it is entirely reasonable and incredibly helpful to seek a second opinion from another specialist. Gathering information from multiple experts can help you consider different perspectives and make a decision that feels thoughtful, informed, and aligned with your goals for treatment.

Choosing the right provider is an important part of your food allergy journey. Working with a board-certified allergist ensures that you or your child are receiving care from a physician trained specifically in diagnosing and managing allergic conditions. You can search for certified allergists through the American Academy of Allergy, Asthma & Immunology (AAAAI) at www.aaaai.org and the American College of Allergy, Asthma & Immunology (ACAAI) at www.acaai.org.

If you are exploring immunotherapy, such as oral immunotherapy (OIT), a helpful starting point is the Food Allergy Support Team (FAST) website at www.fastoit.org, which lists providers who offer these specialized treatments. While these resources are not exhaustive, they provide a reliable first step in finding qualified providers to discuss your options and tailor a plan that meets your needs.

A Good Provider/Patient Fit as a Starting Point

By the time oral immunotherapy became a real option for us, I was exhausted. While participating in the peanut patch clinical trial, I searched for OIT providers near Buffalo, New York. Eventually, I found a clinic in Pittsburgh, Pennsylvania, about a four-hour drive each way. Under other circumstances, that distance might have felt unreasonable, but the closest alternative was nearly six hours away in Michigan. Pittsburgh felt comparatively manageable.

My hometown was roughly halfway through the drive, which I hoped would help make the trips more manageable. My mother had been my primary source of support and the only person regularly watching the kids. She lived at the halfway-point of the drive, which made the logistics of treatment feel more realistic.

When I called the clinic, the doctor spent almost an hour on the phone with me. He walked me through how treatment would work, how billing would be handled across state lines, and how our distance from the clinic might affect the pacing of OIT. I explained my son's history in detail, including the patterns that suggested an unusually high level of sensitivity. Instead of minimizing those concerns, he responded with validation and empathy, paired with steady confidence that we could still pursue OIT safely by moving carefully and slowly.

That phone call represented renewed hope for us. It lifted me out of a level of fear and anxiety that had begun to feel constant and replaced it with a calm sense of confidence that this was the next right step. We had been hesitant to walk away from the opportunity to complete the peanut patch trial, but the trust I felt with this doctor outweighed that uncertainty. Taking the leap required a fair amount of coordination on my end, yet the immediate rapport with this provider made it feel manageable.

At that point, my son was only five. He was surprisingly open to the idea of changing paths, though he asked if he could meet the doctor before we made a final decision. I remember thinking how reasonable and grounded that request was. At our appointment, the doctor was calm, friendly, and reassuring. A part of me still expected him to dismiss the significance of my son's past reactions, but instead he explained very simply how we would approach treatment given his sensitivity. My son felt comfortable with the doctor almost immediately, which made it easier to recognize that this was the next step on our path.

Preparing for a Conversation with a Potential Treatment Provider

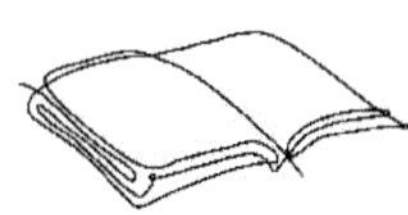 Choosing a doctor is not just about credentials or logistics. It is about finding a guide you trust who listens carefully, explains things clearly, and helps you navigate the road ahead with confidence. Meeting with a specialist can be an opportunity to gather information and better understand what treatment might look like for you or your child.

Some practices may be able to answer your initial questions over the phone to save you time ruling in/out their practice as a possibility. The questions that follow can help to guide the conversations at appointments and ensure you leave with the information you need to make an informed decision. Please feel free to make copies of this page as needed in the event that you are fortunate enough to have multiple options for a possible provider. Hopefully, your doctor will also share handouts and materials that answer many of these questions.

Including Your Child's Perspective

It can also be helpful to pay attention to your child's experience. Of course, we don't want to place the weight of an adult medical decision on a child's shoulders. Choosing a treatment provider is ultimately the responsibility of the parent or caregiver, but including your child's perspective can provide useful information.

Children often notice things adults might overlook, like how comfortable they felt speaking with the doctor, whether the office environment felt welcoming, or whether the experience made them feel more or less anxious about treatment. You may find that your child clearly gravitates toward one office or provider over another. Sometimes this preference will be based on meaningful factors, such as feeling listened to or reassured by the doctor. Other times it may be based on things that are less central to the decision, like video games in the waiting room or the clinic being located near a favorite store or restaurant. Their feedback doesn't have to determine the decision, but it can be a valuable piece of information as you consider the overall experience.

New Provider Appointment

Provider Information

Practice / Clinic Name: ___________________________

Provider(s) Name(s): ___________________________

Board-Certified Allergist:	Yes / No

Years in Practice: ___________________________

Experience with Treatment: ___________________________

Clinic Location (s): ___________________________

____

____

____

Phone / Contact: ___________________________

Website: ___________________________

Social Media: ___________________________

Logistics

Distance from Home: ___________________________

Typical Travel Time: ___________________________

Insurance Accepted:	Yes / No / Unsure

Estimated Out-of-Pocket Costs Discussed: ___________________________

____

____

____

____

____

Treatments Offered

Oral Immunotherapy (OIT):	Yes / No

Sublingual Immunotherapy (SLIT):	Yes / No

Subcutaneous Immunotherapy (SCIT):	Yes / No

Biologic Medications (e.g., adjunct therapy):	Yes / No

Other Treatments Offered: ___________________________

Treatment Options

Which treatment options do you think might be appropriate in our situation and why?

____

____

____

Treatment Process

What does the treatment schedule typically look like in the beginning?

____
____
____

How often are visits to the clinic typically required?

____
____
____

What should we expect during dose increases or monitoring visits?

____
____
____

How do you handle reactions if they occur?

____
____
____

Safety and Monitoring

How do we contact the clinic if we have concerns between visits?

____
____
____

What are your procedures for symptoms and reactions outside of the office?

____
____
____

Other Topics Discussed

____
____
____

Personal Reflection

After your conversation, take a moment to reflect on the following, or any other aspects of your experience: Did I feel heard and respected during this conversation? Were my questions answered clearly? Does this provider's approach feel like a good fit for our family?

____
____
____

Questions to Ask or Observe About Your Child's Experience

How did my child seem during the visit?
Calm / Nervous / Curious / Overwhelmed / Other____

How did the provider and staff interact with my child?

____
____
____

How did my child speak to/interact with the office and staff?

____
____
____

Questions to ask your child:

What did you think about today?

____
____
____

What parts of today did you like, and were there any you didn't like?

____
____
____

What questions do you have about the things we talked about today?

____
____
____

Final Reflection: Choosing the Right Guide for Your Journey

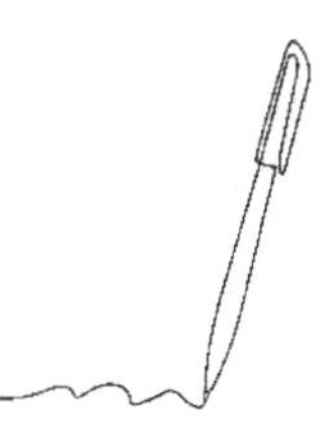

After meeting with providers, it can be helpful to pause and reflect on the overall picture. No doctor will be perfect in every category, and in some cases your options may be limited by geography, insurance, or availability. But when multiple factors are considered together, families often find that one option begins to feel like the clearer fit.

Use the space below and the prompts to compare/contrast and organize your thoughts.

Trust and Communication

Which providers listened carefully to my questions and concerns? Whose explanations make sense to me? With whom did I feel comfortable asking follow-up questions?

____

____

Experience and Approach

Which providers have experience with the treatment(s) we are considering? Whose approaches to treatment align with our goals and comfort level? Who explained both benefits and risks clearly?

____

____

Practical Considerations

Which locations are manageable for the distance and frequency of visits required? Do the financial aspects feel clear and feasible? Which programs/approaches seem realistic for daily life?

____

____

Overall Fit

Which practice(s) felt organized, supportive, and responsive? Which provider(s) seem best equipped and experienced to manage the ups and downs? Where did I/my child feel comfortable/cared for?

____

____

My Overall Impression (consider yourself fortunate if you find more than one good option!)

____

____

____

Finding Mental Health Support

 Food allergy treatment often brings up fear, uncertainty, hypervigilance, grief, medical trauma, family stress, and nervous system overwhelm. Therapy can be an important part of your care team, not because something is "wrong" or you "need" it, but because this experience is challenging on many levels and support can be helpful.

One of the best places to start is often with your medical team. Ask your allergist or primary care provider if they have local therapists they regularly refer patients to. They often know which clinicians understand medical anxiety, chronic illness, and the emotional side of managing complex health conditions. They may also have personal experience collaborating with those therapists and know who tends to be a good fit for families navigating food allergy treatment.

What To Look For
Finding a therapist with personal experience in food allergy or immunotherapy can be wonderful, but it is also rare and not necessarily the most important factor. What often matters more is finding someone with strong training and experience in trauma-informed care.

Many people are surprised to learn that not all therapists are specifically trained to work with trauma. A therapist may be excellent in general mental health care and still have limited experience helping people process medical trauma, nervous system dysregulation, or chronic states of fear and hypervigilance. Because food allergy experiences often involve emergency situations, unpredictability, repeated stress, and a body that has learned to stay on high alert, trauma-informed care can make a significant difference.

A good therapist does not need to be a food allergy specialist to help you. They do need to be curious, collaborative, and able to respect the reality of the medical risk without minimizing it or pathologizing appropriate caution. A good therapist should help you feel safer, not dismissed or more afraid.

Food allergy anxiety is different from many other anxiety presentations because the risk is real. The goal is not to convince you that danger does not exist. The goal is to help you find regulation, flexibility, and trust while still respecting legitimate safety needs.

Be cautious of anyone who immediately treats your anxiety like something to simply "get over" or encourages unsafe exposure without understanding the medical context. You want someone who can hold both truths at once: Yes, there is real risk, and yes, you may benefit from support around how your nervous system responds to that risk.

It is also important to notice how a therapist responds when they do not know something. They do not need to know everything about food allergies on day one. What matters more is whether they respond with curiosity rather than defensiveness. Helpful therapists say things like, "Help me understand what feels hardest here," or "What does safety look like for you?" Less helpful therapists minimize, dismiss, or assume they already understand.

Finally, fit matters. Therapy is relational. Credentials matter, and so does connection. Do you feel understood? Do you feel judged? Do you leave feeling clearer or more overwhelmed? Do you feel like you have to defend, justify, or overexplain your experience?

The right fit often feels less like "they have all the answers" and more like "I feel safe enough to do this work here."

You are allowed to ask your therapist questions, get information about their experience and qualifications, and express your preferences for what your work together might look like.

This is not about finding the perfect therapist. It is about finding someone who feels safe enough, skilled enough, and collaborative enough to walk this part of the road with you.

New Mental Health Provider Appointment

Practice / Clinic Name: _____________________________

Provider Name(s): _____________________________

Location: _____________________________

Phone/Contact: _____________________________

Website: _____________________________

Referred By (Allergist, PCP, Friend, School, Other): ______________________

Credentials:

☐ Psychologist ☐ LCSW ☐ LMHC, LPC, LMFT ☐ Other: ____________

Specialized Training in Trauma: ☐ Yes ☐ No

Experience with Medical Anxiety, Chronic Illness, or Food Allergies: ☐ Yes ☐ No

Logistics

Appointment Type: ☐ In-Person ☐ Virtual ☐ Both/Combination

Insurance Accepted: ☐ Yes ☐ No ☐ Unsure

Distance from Home: _____________________________

Typical Travel Time: _____________________________

Estimated Out-of-Pocket Costs Discussed: ______________________

Days/Times for Appointments: __________________________

Waitlist Length (if applicable): __________________________

Areas of Support

Individual Therapy for Parent: ☐ Yes ☐ No

Individual Therapy for Child: ☐ Yes ☐ No

Family Therapy: ☐ Yes ☐ No

Support for Medical and Health Anxiety: ☐ Yes ☐ No

Specific Training and Experience with Trauma: ☐ Yes ☐ No

Support for Needle Fear / Procedure Anxiety: ☐ Yes ☐ No

Other Areas of Support Offered: ________________________

Understanding Their Approach

How do you approach anxiety when the risk involved is real, such as food allergy or medical concerns?

____

____

How do you work with trauma, nervous system regulation, or medical stress?

How do you involve parents or caregivers when working with children?

What does support typically look like during high-stress medical situations or treatment transitions?

If you are not familiar with food allergy treatment, how do you approach learning about a family's specific experience?

Safety and Communication

How do we contact you between sessions if concerns come up?

What does support look like during a crisis, major reaction, or difficult medical event?

How do you coordinate care with allergists, pediatricians, or other providers if needed?

Personal Reflection

After your conversation, take a moment to reflect on the following:

Did I feel heard and respected during this conversation?

Were my concerns taken seriously?

Did this provider understand the difference between appropriate caution and anxiety taking over?

____

____

Did they seem curious and open, or dismissive and minimizing?

____

____

Does this provider's approach feel like a good fit for me or my family?

____

____

Questions to Ask or Observe About Your Child's Experience (if the appointment involved your child)

How did my child seem during the visit?

____

____

How did the therapist and staff interact with my child?

____

____

How did my child respond to the office, therapist, and overall environment?

____

____

Did my child seem emotionally safe enough to participate honestly?

____

____

Questions to Ask Your Child

What did you think about today?

____

____

What parts of today did you like, and were there any you didn't like?

____

____

What questions do you have about the things we talked about today?

____

____

Chapter 4:
Shared Decisions Within Your Family

Involving Your Child in Decision-Making

 Once you've explored treatment options and discussed them with your healthcare team, the next step is thinking about your child's role in the decision-making process. Involving your child thoughtfully can increase their sense of autonomy, reduce anxiety, and help them feel respected. This works best when you, as parents or caregivers, have already clarified the options among yourselves.

Going through the decision-making process with all adults involved first ensures you can present a clear, honest plan to your child without raising hopes about options that may not be feasible due to medical, logistical, or personal reasons.

Engaging Your Child with the Doctor

Depending on your child's personality, it may be important they hear directly from the allergist whether they are a good candidate for treatment and which options the doctor recommends. Many allergists will naturally and appropriately include children in the conversation. You may choose to have another adult join you for appointments to entertain your child while you speak to the doctor alone about options. Either way, the conversation should be an ongoing discussion that welcomes questions and concerns and translates medical information into terms they can understand.

Respecting Your Child's Voice

Sometimes, a child may give a firm "no" to a treatment idea. This deserves attention before other factors are considered. It's important to explore whether their resistance is based on fear, misunderstanding, or other personal reasons. If your child continues to resist despite encouragement, a collaborative conversation can help. Allergy clinic staff or a trained therapist can support this process by helping the child articulate their feelings, understand their concerns, and gain insight into their perspective.

Common Fears and Misunderstandings

Some children refuse oral immunotherapy because they believe it will involve frequent use of epinephrine or repeated trips to the emergency room. Fear of reactions, injections, ambulance rides, or ER visits is often rooted in past experiences or uncertainty about the treatment. Preparing to address these fears directly can help your child feel safer and more informed. You'll want to be ready to explain the realities of dosing, reaction management, and emergency use of epinephrine. By addressing their questions and fears up front and including their goals in decision-making, you create a foundation for honest dialogue and treatment success. Once your child feels informed and heard, they are more likely to engage openly in the decision-making process.

Several activities to support conversations with your child about immunotherapy are included below. These are not meant to be used all at once, but rather as tools to guide an ongoing, gradual conversation over time.

Magic Wand Exercise (Explanation)

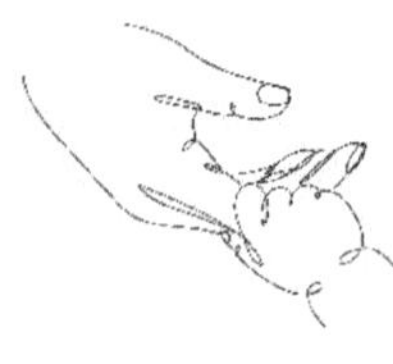

This exercise is a useful way to support your child anytime they are experiencing frustration, fear, sadness, or difficult emotions. I recommend using this to start a general conversation about allergy management before discussing specific treatments. *Note:* Bookmark this page for use as a general exercise anytime your child is having a difficult time, not just when making treatment decisions.

About the Magic Wand Exercise

Do you ever catch yourself in child-like fantasies of having a fairy godmother show up and solve your problems, finding a genie in a bottle, or winning the lottery? Most adults and children experience some form of wishful thinking like this occasionally.

Wishful thinking is not denial or avoidance. It is a natural mental process that helps us express unmet needs, longings, and emotions, especially when situations feel out of our control. When we allow ourselves to imagine what we wish were different, we are often revealing something important about what we need most right now, such as safety, reassurance, rest, or understanding. Naming these wishes does not mean we expect them to come true exactly as imagined. In fact, we usually wish for things because we know that they aren't possible, and that impossibility feels unfair or frustrating.

Wishful thinking gives our nervous system a sense of being heard and acknowledged, steering us away from our tendency to suppress or ignore uncomfortable thoughts and feelings that can't be resolved. This can reduce emotional pressure and make it easier to cope with what is actually happening, even when the circumstances themselves cannot change.

The magic wand activity uses imagination to give voice to wishes, needs, and feelings that may be hard to say out loud. Instead of problem-solving right away, we pause and imagine what we wish could be different. This is not about pretending everything is fine or avoiding reality. It is about letting the nervous system experience being heard, understood, and cared for.

Why This Works

When we imagine receiving comfort, safety, or support, the brain and nervous system respond as if some of that care is happening in real time. This can reduce stress, soften big emotions, and help us access feelings that are otherwise stuck or overwhelming.

For children especially, imagination is often safer and more accessible than direct conversation. It feels like play and allows them to have control or lead the conversation. When doing this activity with a child, allow yourself to fully enter the fantasy with them. Follow their lead and get curious about the details. Ask gentle questions about what the place looks like, sounds like, smells like, or feels like in their body. Notice the colors, the temperature, the textures, and who or what is there with them. The more sensory detail the child adds, the more real and regulating the experience becomes for their nervous system. Invite your child to draw their vision or think of a song that represents it to help you remember this imagined place together and gently bring it back during moments of stress. A simple reminder such as "Do you remember your magic wand place?" or playing the song they chose can help the child access a familiar sense of safety and comfort, even when things feel hard.

For teens and adults, it can bypass overthinking or suppression and allow deeper emotional truth to surface. When using this exercise, be especially careful not to correct, interpret, or turn the fantasy into a lesson or lecture. Instead, meet the imagination with curiosity and respect. Listen for any details that reveal how they want to feel. Some may describe their wish in images or metaphors rather than full stories. Others may keep it brief. Both are valid. You can gently reflect what you hear and, if invited, ask about sensory details such as what feels calmer in their body or what the space around them is like in the imagined moment. Over time, you can reference this imagined experience in a low-key way during stressful moments, offering it as a coping option rather than a directive. This preserves autonomy while still providing emotional support and continuity.

With children of any age, this exercise also supports co-regulation. Being witnessed in our wishes, without immediately fixing or correcting them, helps build trust and emotional safety. Having something to "do" to support our children can move us out of our tendency to want to solve their problems for them, and allows us to be present with them and validate their emotions and experience.

The magic wand activity is not about pretending that medical realities will disappear, ignoring safety guidelines, or replacing professional care. It is also not about forcing positive thinking or convincing yourself or your child that everything is fine when it is not. Wishful thinking, in this context, is not meant to change outcomes. It is meant to change how alone or overwhelmed the experience feels. By separating emotional needs from problem-solving, we allow space for feelings to be expressed without immediately needing to fix them. This often makes it easier to return to practical decision-making with more clarity and steadiness.

Closing The Activity or Conversation

The most difficult part of this exercise is usually the natural desire to want to conclude with a promise, a solution, or a plan. As adults, we often feel an urge to reassure by saying what we will do differently, what will improve, or how we will make sure the wish comes true.

While this instinct comes from care, it can sometimes pull us out of the emotional moment too quickly. The purpose of this activity is not to create an action step. It is to let the wish exist and be witnessed. When we rush to fix, promise, or problem-solve, the nervous system may miss the experience of simply being heard.

Instead of closing with a promise or a plan, try closing with presence, validation, and connection.

*An audio version of this activity is available for free on the *Don't Feed the Fear* podcast. You can find the "Bonus Meditation: Magic Wand" exercise anywhere you get your podcasts.

The Magic Wand Exercise

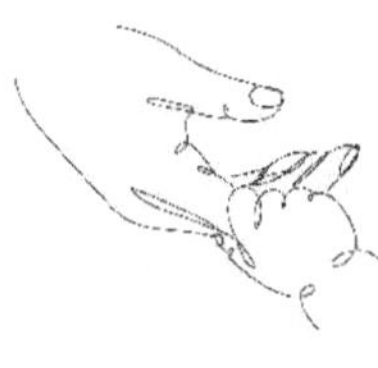 Children don't always have the words to directly express their fears, frustrations, or longings. This is especially true when it comes to something as complex as food allergies or medical treatment. The "magic wand" exercise is a simple way to gently open that door. Remember: this activity is not about fixing, solving, or correcting. It is about listening, validating, and connecting.

Introduce the Exercise

"If I had a magic wand and could do or change anything for you, anything at all, what would you wish for?"

Let your child know there are no limits and no "right" answers.

Follow Their Lead

Once your child shares their wish, stay curious. You can gently explore by asking questions like:

- "What would that be like?"

- "What would feel different if that happened?"

- "What would you notice first?"

- "What would be easier?"

- "Who else would notice?"

Let them describe the experience in as much detail as they want. Some children will share a lot, others only a little. Both are okay.

Listen, Reflect, and Stay With Them

Your most important job is to *be with them*, not to fix it. You might reflect back what you hear:

- "That sounds really important to you."

- "I can see how much you wish for that."

- "That makes a lot of sense."

Try to avoid:

- Explaining why it can't happen

- Reassuring too quickly

- Turning it into a lesson or solution

Their wish will probably be something impossible, and it is still meaningful. It is a window into their internal world.

As Big Feelings Come Up

Your child might feel sad, frustrated, or quiet. This is not a problem to solve. Stay grounded and reassure them:

- "I'm really glad you told me."

- "I'm here with you."

- "That's a big feeling."

Being present, calm, and attuned is the most regulating thing you can offer.

For You (Parent Reflection)

After the conversation, take a moment to reflect:

- What did your child's wish tell you about their experience?

- Did anything surprise you?

- What emotions came up for you as you listened?

You don't need to act on this immediately. Just noticing is enough.

Closing the Exercise

There is no need to tie this up neatly.

You might simply say:

"Thank you for telling me. I'm really glad I got to hear that."

As the activity ends, give your child space to process. Stay gently present and follow their lead by offering physical comfort, quiet proximity, or a bit of distance, depending on what they seem to need in that moment.

Jot down anything you'd like to remember from this exercise:

____
____
____
____
____
____
____

Explaining Immunotherapy to Children

 Before we explain immunotherapy to a child, it is important to make sure they understand what an allergy is in the first place. You might begin by explaining that everyone has an immune system that protects us from germs and things that can truly make us sick. Most of the time it keeps us healthy, but sometimes it gets confused.

With a food allergy, the immune system misreads a regular food as if it were a dangerous invader. Instead of recognizing it as harmless, it sounds the alarm and launches an attack. That attack creates the symptoms that we call an allergic reaction.

Immunotherapy is a way of teaching the immune system a new story. It slowly and carefully shows the immune system that the food is not actually dangerous. Over time, the immune system can learn to respond more calmly. Instead of sounding the alarm and attacking, it begins to recognize the food and stand down.

At any age, the goal is the same. We are not telling children their body is broken or bad. We are explaining that the immune system got confused. Immunotherapy is not about forcing their body to do something scary. It is about teaching it, slowly and safely, to recognize what is actually dangerous and what is not.

Immunotherapy is a commitment. For many families, it's a hopeful one. When explained in developmentally appropriate, honest ways, children are remarkably capable of understanding that their bodies are learning something new.

Remember to only explain the options your doctor has offered and confirmed are available and medically appropriate for your child. Trying to cover all possibilities can cause unnecessary confusion, excitement, or worry. Verify with your allergist which options are appropriate before discussing them with your child. If your child will attend an appointment where multiple treatment options may be discussed, consider having another adult with you who can stay with your child in the waiting area to prevent overwhelm and confusion.

General Tips for All Ages
1. Use simple, concrete language and check for understanding.
2. Frame doses and treatments as steps on the journey, not as risky or scary events.
3. Normalize curiosity, questions, and complex feelings about the process.
4. Keep explanations aligned with what their doctor has approved so expectations match the reality of what is offered.
5. Reinforce safety and support: "You are never alone. Mom, Dad, and the doctors are your guides."
6. Include discussion of concrete goals and reasons treatment may be helpful and beneficial.

Introducing Immunotherapy as a Journey

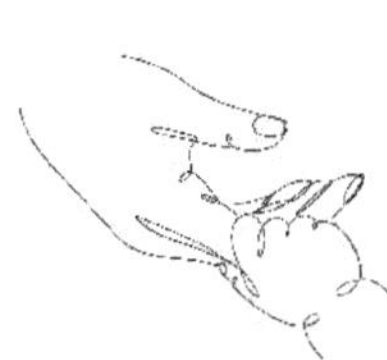

Framing immunotherapy as a journey is a helpful metaphor that can foster understanding and curiosity, rather than anxiety or fear. Just like any journey, there are steps to take, tools to carry, and guides to help along the way. The goal is to help your child understand that they will gradually build their body's "skills" to handle allergens safely, and that you and their care team will be traveling alongside them the whole time.

Having a general conversation about immunotherapy allows time for your child to understand that concept before discussing the details of specific treatment options. Children tend to receive information best when it is shared throughout small conversations over time, rather than one long, serious discussion.

Preschool (Under 5)

- Focus on: Small steps, playful language, reassurance, and routine.
- Key idea: The body can learn something different a little bit at a time.
- Example introduction:
  "We're going on a little adventure to help your body learn how to handle your allergen(s) safely. Every day we'll take tiny steps to teach your body something new."
- Emphasize that they are safe, that you are with them, and that each small step is a success.

Elementary (Ages 5–10)

- Focus on: Cause-and-effect, agency, and understanding progress.
- Key idea: The immune system can learn not to react with repeated practice.
- Example introduction:
  "We're starting a journey to help your body learn not to react to your allergen(s). Each dose is like training your body to know what's safe, like practicing climbing a hill until it feels easier. We'll go step by step, and you'll notice how your body learns along the way."
- Encourage questions and help them track milestones, reinforcing the idea of progress along the journey.

Preteens / Teens / Adolescents

- Focus on: Independence, understanding strategy, and self-monitoring.
- Key idea: They are active participants and responsible for part of their journey.
- Example introduction:
  "We're beginning a journey to help your body learn to tolerate your allergen(s) safely. You'll be paying attention to how you feel and making decisions with guidance, like navigating a trail with a map and compass. Every step you take decreases your reactivity."
- Highlight that the child's personal goals will be central, mistakes or adjustments are normal on any journey, and that you and the care team are there as guides.

Checking In With Your Child About the Journey

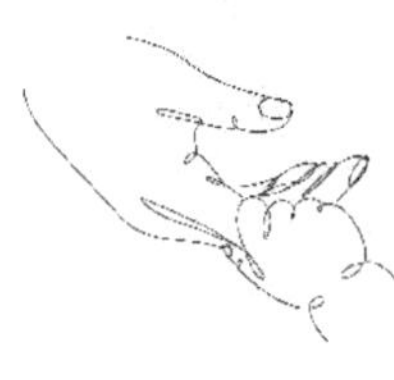 This is a discussion guide to use after you've introduced the idea of immunotherapy as a journey to your child and shared details about the specific treatment(s) you are considering. Refer back to the earlier sections of this workbook for guidance and sample language for each treatment. It's important to pause and involve your child in reflecting on what they've learned, what questions they have, and how they feel to help them feel heard and actively involved.

Note: Bookmark this page and come back to it throughout treatment. Use it for support anytime there are changes, new doses, challenges, or milestones that should be discussed. Encouraging your child to provide input helps them practice self-advocacy, understand the process, and feel involved in decisions that affect their health.

Guiding the Conversation

- Engage your child in an activity rather than having a formal sit-down conversation. Eating, walking, or doing a hands-on craft or activity may help them be more receptive.
- Explore the child's goals and what may motivate them to complete the treatment. Keep these concrete and age-appropriate, such as foods they may want to try, experiences they want to have, or places they want to go.
- Normalize questions and curiosity: Children may ask about the process or risks. Answer honestly but concisely, emphasizing safety and the journey metaphor: "Each step is a checkpoint on your path."
- Avoid leading questions like, "What are you nervous about?" Mirror your child's words back to them in the conversation wherever possible to show them you understand.

Preschool (Under 5)

- Goal: Encourage curiosity, basic understanding, and expression of feelings
- Sample Questions:
    - Can you tell me what you think this will be like?
    - What parts sound good or interesting to you?
    - What parts aren't you sure about?
    - Do you have any ideas for ways we can make it easier or more fun?
    - If you wanted to explain this to your friend, what would you say?
    - Can we draw or act out what we'll be doing?
    - Who can help us with this journey?

Elementary (Ages 5-10)

- Goal: Support understanding, reasoning, and planning
- Sample Questions:
    - What do you already know about this treatment?
    - What questions do you have?
    - How do you think your body will change or respond along the way?
    - Do you have any ideas for making this a good experience?
    - Who could we ask to help us with this journey?
    - What parts are you excited about? Unsure about? Why?
    - How can we track or celebrate your progress along the journey?

Preteens / Adolescents

- Goal: Promote autonomy, alignment with child's goals, critical thinking, and self-advocacy
- Sample Questions:
    - How do you understand what will happen during your immunotherapy?
    - What worries you, and what excites you about this journey?
    - Are there ways you want to be involved in decisions about dosing or scheduling?
    - How can you monitor how your body responds and let us know?
    - What strategies help you feel prepared or calm when things feel uncertain?
    - Are there questions you want to ask your doctor or care team?
    - How would you explain this journey to someone else your age?

General Tips:

- Give your child space to answer in their own words, and validate their thoughts and feelings.
- Revisit these questions periodically, especially when new challenges or milestones arise.
- Consider journaling together or letting your child express their thoughts and feelings through drawing.
- Encourage your child to keep asking questions as the journey continues. They will come to understand and process more over time than they could initially.

Notes:

____
____
____
____
____
____
____

The Financial Reality of Food Allergy Treatment Decisions

 When families begin exploring immunotherapy, the first question is often medical. Is this safe? Is this right for my child? What are the risks and benefits? Very quickly, another question follows, sometimes quietly and sometimes with urgency. Can we afford this? The financial cost of food allergy treatment is real, significant, and often unpredictable.

Unlike many medical interventions, immunotherapy is not a single procedure with a clear price tag. It is a process that unfolds over many months or years, with costs that vary widely depending on the clinic, the type of treatment, insurance coverage, geographic location, and individual medical needs. Many find themselves trying to make sense of incomplete information. Coverage may change and estimates may shift. Some costs are known upfront, while others emerge only as treatment progresses. It is common to feel uneasy committing when the financial impact is not fully clear. That uncertainty can activate stress, anxiety, and pressure to make the "right" decision quickly.

When financial stress is layered on top of medical risk and fear, it can affect how clearly we think, how regulated we feel, and how supported we feel throughout the treatment process. For some, the cost feels manageable but requires planning. For others, it feels overwhelming or impossible without significant sacrifice. Many patients and families hold complicated feelings at the same time, hope for freedom from food anxiety alongside worry about long-term financial impact.

Financial considerations are not separate from emotional readiness or treatment success. They influence stress levels, family dynamics, consistency with appointments and dosing, and patients' and parents' ability to stay regulated when challenges arise. This is why it is important to talk openly about money in the context of food allergy care.

The next page is designed to help you organize the financial pieces of the treatment(s) you are considering. It will not produce an exact number or a final decision. Instead, it offers a way to anticipate categories of cost, identify unknowns, and prepare questions for your medical team and insurance provider. Even partial clarity can reduce stress and increase a sense of control.

As you move through these exercises, you will be reminded that the cost of treatment is not only financial. There are other expenses that do not show up on a bill but still require energy, time, flexibility, and emotional bandwidth. These include the cost of missed work or school, the mental load of planning and monitoring, the impact on siblings, the strain on relationships, and the cumulative stress of living in a state of vigilance. You may not be able to anticipate them all, and naming them does not mean treatment is not worth pursuing. It means acknowledging the full picture. When families are supported in seeing both the visible and invisible costs of care, they are better able to make decisions that are sustainable, compassionate, and aligned with their values.

Estimating the Financial Cost of Food Allergy Immunotherapy

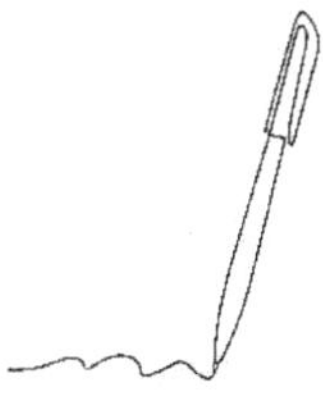

Immunotherapy costs can vary widely based on provider, location, insurance coverage, length of treatment, and individual medical needs. Most families are not able to calculate an exact total cost upfront, and that is normal.

The goals of this exercise are to help you:

- Anticipate categories of expenses

- Reduce financial surprises

- Clarify questions to ask your allergist and insurance provider

- Consider the emotional impact of financial stress alongside medical decision-making

You may not be able to fill in every box with certainty. Estimates, ranges, and notes are still helpful. Consider throughout what may be weekly/monthly/yearly patterns rather than one-time expenses.

Treatment-related medical costs (direct cost of care)

Estimated costs to explore or record:
Initial consultation and evaluation fees
Food challenges or baseline testing
Labwork/testing fees (skin or blood tests)
Medications
Enrollment or program fees
Dosing visits or supervised up-dosing appointments
Maintenance visit costs

Notes and questions:

Insurance and Out-of-Pocket Considerations

Insurance-related factors to consider:
Deductible amount and whether it has been met
Co-pays or co-insurance per visit
Coverage for food challenges or procedures
Coverage differences for in- and out-of-network providers
Dose, pharmacy, or compounding costs, if applicable

Notes and questions:

____

____

Non-Medical and Hidden Costs

Travel costs/mileage

Parking or tolls

Time off work or reduced work hours

Additional childcare costs

Meals or snacks during trips/long appointments

Lodging (if traveling long distances)

Notes and questions:

____

____

Emotional and Cognitive Costs

Financial stress affects the nervous system and decision-making. This section invites reflection, not judgment.

Consider the following questions:

- How does financial uncertainty affect my stress level?

- Does financial strain increase anxiety around treatment decisions?

- Are there worries about affordability that I am carrying silently?

- How does financial pressure impact our family dynamics or relationships?

These responses matter. Financial stress is a real part of treatment readiness.

Notes and questions:

____

____

Offsetting and Support Options

Payment plans through the clinic (uncommon)   ________________________________

Flexible spending or health savings accounts   ________________________________

Employer benefits or medical leave options   ________________________________

Extended family support   ________________________________

Grants, scholarships, or advocacy organization resources   ________________________________

Adjusting timelines to reduce financial pressure   ________________________________

Notes and questions:

____

____

Big Picture Reflection

What feels manageable right now?

____

____

What feels overwhelming?

____

____

What additional information would help you feel more grounded in this decision?

____

____

There is no "right" answer. This exercise is about clarity and self-compassion.

Important Reminder

This workbook is designed to support important conversations with your allergist, clinic billing staff, and insurance provider. Financial planning is part of medical care, and it is appropriate to ask detailed questions before beginning treatment.

My Treatment Comparison Chart

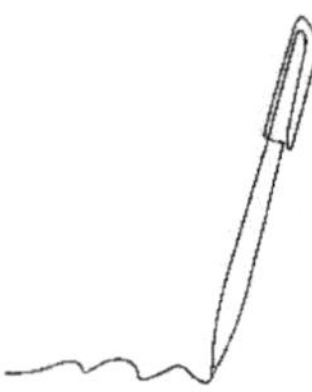

Fill in the chart below for any treatment options you are considering. Add any thoughts, observations, or information that you want to consider. Use the questions on the following page as prompts.

Treatment Option	Potential Benefits	Possible Drawbacks or Challenges	Practical Barriers	Questions I Still Have
Sublingual Immunotherapy (SLIT)				
Oral Immunotherapy (OIT)				
Tolerance Induction Program (TIP)				
Biologic Medications				
Careful Avoidance				

Are there any risks/benefits to waiting rather than pursuing treatment now?

____

____

What impact might this have on short- and long-term safety?

____

____

What side effects, lifestyle adjustments, or uncertainties concern me?

____

____

What considerations for each treatment are important regarding access to providers, travel, insurance coverage, costs, time commitment, waiting list for availability?

____

____

What aspects of different approaches are aligned or misaligned with my values and priorities?

____

____

What mental health factors are impacting my decision (social impact, anxiety levels, lifestyle restrictions, and accidental exposure risk)?

____

____

Am I considering treatment for a single food or multiple and how does that impact my choice?

____

____

Reflecting on Your Responses

What themes do you notice in your responses? Are there options that feel more aligned with your medical needs, values, lifestyle, financial means, or comfort level?

____

____

Which factors matter most in your decision-making right now? (Examples: safety, quality of life, financial cost, time commitment, or emotional readiness)

____

____

What questions do you want to discuss with your allergist or care team?

____

____

Clarifying Your Choice and Feeling Confident in It

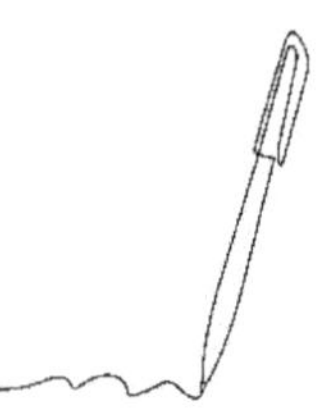

This exercise is designed to help you feel confident, intentional, and at peace with your decision, while also identifying when you might choose to revisit the conversation and reconsider this choice in the future.

My Reasons Right Now

List your decision and the reasons that it feels right for you or your family at this time. What factors influenced your decision? What concerns, limitations, or priorities are important right now?

____
____
____
____
____

What This Decision Supports

Every decision supports something. What does this choice make easier, safer, or more manageable right now? Consider emotional well-being, daily routines, financial considerations, medical factors, and family needs.

____
____
____
____
____

Addressing Doubt and Outside Pressure

What thoughts or worries come up about this decision? Common examples are: _Am I doing enough?_, _What if I regret this?_, _Should I be doing more?_ Write them down and then gently respond to those thoughts with what you know to be true:

____
____
____
____
____

Confidence Statement

I am choosing to pursue this treatment OR I am choosing not to pursue treatment right now because…

____
____
____
____

 I feel confident in this decision because…

____
____
____
____

AND/OR
I don't feel confident in this decision because...
Here are the reasons why and the steps I can take to be more sure:

____
____
____
____

When Might I Revisit This?

This is not about second-guessing your decision. It is about creating clarity for the future.

You might revisit this decision if a new treatment becomes available, you feel more ready, your child is older, your circumstances or capacity change, or you receive new medical information. There is no way to know for sure when or why this might be, but explore what factors might lead you to reconsider your choices.

____
____
____
____

Closing Reflection

I can make thoughtful decisions and adjust them over time. I don't need to have everything decided forever.

Parent & Caregiver Alignment

 One of the most important and often overlooked parts of preparing for treatment is not medical, but relational. Food allergy management already requires coordination between caregivers. Beginning immunotherapy, or any new treatment approach, increases that need.

Dosing schedules, safety protocols, symptom interpretation, and emotional responses all become shared responsibilities during treatment. When caregivers are not aligned, even small differences in approach can create confusion, tension, or inconsistency that affects both the child's experience and treatment outcomes. Alignment does not mean complete agreement on every detail. It means that the adults involved in a child's care have had the opportunity to understand the options, express their concerns, and move toward a shared plan that feels informed and intentional.

It is very common for caregivers to have different emotional reactions to treatment decisions. One may feel hopeful and ready to move forward. Another may feel hesitant, protective, or overwhelmed by the risks. Each perspective can reflect a different aspect of care: safety, quality of life, long-term goals, or emotional readiness.

When these perspectives are not discussed openly, they tend to show up indirectly. This can look like second-guessing decisions, inconsistency with protocols, or tension during moments of stress. Children are highly attuned to these dynamics. Even when nothing is said directly, they can sense when the adults around them are not on the same page.

Taking time to align is especially important in families where children move between multiple households or caregiving environments. Consistency across settings helps children feel safe and reduces confusion about expectations. When this is not possible, clarity and communication become even more important.

If you are navigating this decision with another caregiver, consider this an essential part of the process rather than an optional step. The goal is not to rush toward agreement, but to build a shared understanding of what you are choosing and why.

Getting on the Same Page

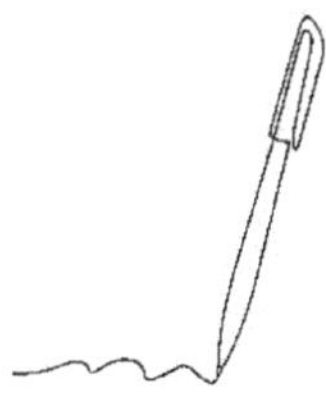

Complete together or separately and then discuss your responses. After discussing together, consider whether there are other important adults in your child's life who may be providing care and need to be on board with the treatment such as grandparents or close friends.

Your Perspective

What feels most important to you about your child's allergy care right now?
What are your biggest hopes if treatment goes well?
What concerns or fears are hardest to ignore?

____
____
____
____

Step 2: Your Decision Lens

What are the most important factors influencing your perspective?
(safety, quality of life, convenience/logistics, emotional impact, long-term outcomes)

____
____
____
____

Readiness Check

On a scale from 1–10, how ready do you feel to begin treatment?
What would help move you one point closer to feeling ready?
What information or experience might make you feel less likely to move forward?

____
____
____
____

Discuss

Set aside time to share your responses. As you talk, listen without interrupting, reflect back what you hear before responding, notice where you already agree.

Where are we aligned?
Where do we feel different, and why?
What information do we still need?
What would help both of us feel more confident moving forward?

____
____
____
____

For Families with Multiple Households or Care Settings

If your child spends time in more than one home or with multiple caregivers:

- Share written treatment plans across all settings

- Clarify who is responsible for dosing, monitoring, and communication

- Agree on how symptoms will be handled and when to use emergency medication

- Keep communication simple, consistent, and documented when possible

Plan:

____
____
____
____
____
____
____
____
____
____

The Sibling Experience

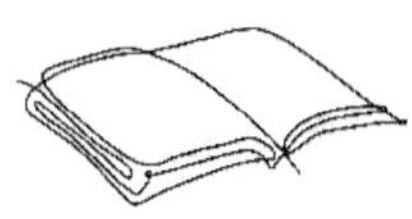 When a child has food allergies, the entire family adapts. Siblings often learn early how to read labels, avoid certain foods, and follow safety rules. They may attend appointments, hear conversations about risk, and witness reactions or close calls. When treatment begins, sibling experiences can shift in ways that are both visible and subtle.

Some siblings feel excited about the possibility of more freedom, while others feel confused when foods that were once "dangerous" are suddenly being used in treatment. Some may feel left out of the attention and care their sibling receives, while others may take on a protective role, becoming highly aware of safety and responsibility. Some may feel many or all of these things at once.

Research shows that healthy siblings of children with chronic illnesses may experience increased levels of anxiety, emotional distress, and feelings of neglect or invisibility, particularly when family attention and resources are, understandably, directed toward the child with medical needs. At the same time, some siblings demonstrate positive adaptations, such as increased empathy, maturity, and resilience. Outcomes for siblings are closely tied to family communication, emotional support, and opportunities for inclusion (Quintana Mariñez et al., 2022).

In the context of food allergy treatment decisions, this highlights the importance of acknowledging siblings' experiences, creating space for their feelings, and involving them appropriately in family discussions to support overall family well-being. They need honest, developmentally appropriate conversations about what is changing, what is staying the same, and what their role is within it. Without this, they may fill in the gaps with their own assumptions, which can lead to confusion, worry, or resentment.

Including siblings in small, meaningful ways can help them feel connected rather than sidelined. This might look like giving them a role in routines, inviting their questions, or simply making space to check in with them individually.

It is also important to recognize that siblings may carry their own version of anxiety. Watching a brother or sister go through treatment can be both reassuring and stressful. They may need support in understanding what is happening and what it means for them. Just like the child in treatment, siblings are adjusting to changing routines.

Sibling Check-In

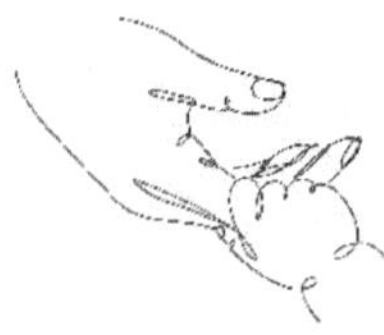 This activity will help you explore siblings' thoughts and feelings about treatment. Encourage them to draw, write, or simply discuss these questions aloud with you. Do this with each sibling individually without the allergic child(ren) present to encourage honest answers and a focus on the sibling's experience and emotions.

What I Know

What do you know about your sibling's allergies?

____

____

What do you know about the treatment they'll be doing?

____

____

What I Wonder

What questions do you have?

____

____

Is there anything that feels confusing or different?

____

____

Check, draw, write, or discuss any feelings about the allergies and/or treatment:

☐ Curious   ☐ Excited   ☐ Worried   ☐ Confused

☐ Left out   ☐ Proud   ☐ Something else: _______________________

Parents/caregivers, respond by:

- Clarifying misunderstandings in simple language
- Reinforcing safety rules that still apply
- Explaining what is changing and what is not
- Acknowledging and validating feelings *without correcting them*

Your Role on the Team

Siblings can feel included by giving them a defined role, if they are interested. Let them choose their role and remind them they are part of the process too.

(Parents, ensure that roles are age-appropriate and that the sibling is not taking on responsibility for safety. The focus should be on support and team-building, not replacing adult care.)

☐ "Food Taster" (tasting doses along with the allergic child)

☐ "Cheerleader" (finding positive things and helping to celebrate them)

☐ "Distraction Expert" (keeping things light or entertaining sibling during dosing time)

☐ "Support Buddy" (offering encouragement by listening, giving hugs, keeping company)

☐ Other

____

____

Caregiver Reflection/Summary

How has this experience impacted my other children?

____

____

Have I made space for their questions and feelings?

____

____

What small step could I take to include or support them more?

____

____

Plan for monitoring and addressing sibling experience throughout treatment:

____

____

____

____

Part IV
Planning the Trip

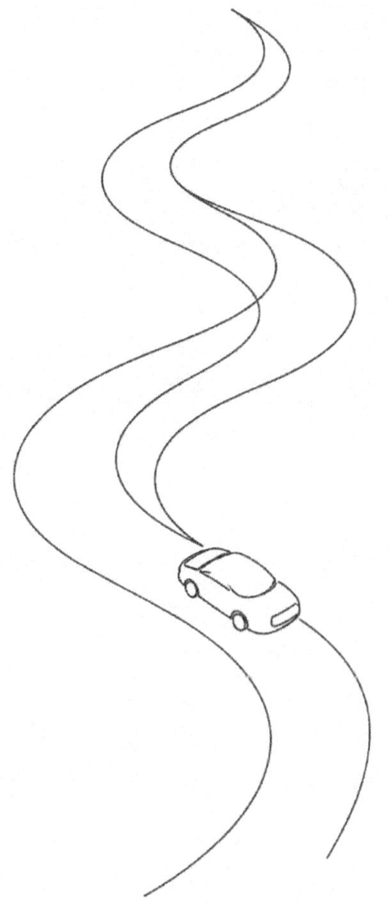

The best way to predict the future
is to create it.

— Unknown

Chapter 5:
Medical Tests and Procedures

As you move from learning about treatment options into choosing a path forward, there's often a subtle but important shift that begins to happen. The details of how to make it work and worries about how it will go can flood patients and parents. Preparation isn't only about logistics or medical readiness. It's also about understanding what this next phase may ask of you and your family, and beginning to orient yourselves to that reality.

For many, this stage brings a mix of clarity, anticipation, and vulnerability. Even when a decision feels right, stepping toward treatment can stir up new questions, old fears, and practical concerns. In the sections that follow, we'll begin to break down the medical, emotional, and day-to-day preparations that are important and often not discussed.

Laying The Medical Groundwork

Moving from considering immunotherapy to actively preparing for it can sometimes feel heavy and complex. There are appointments, tests, food challenges, logistics, and emotions layered into every step. For many, it feels like a daunting process. In episode 72 of the *Don't Feed the Fear* podcast, Dr. Dave Stukus shared a powerful reminder that immunotherapy protocols are built from research models that guide us, but they are not rigid scripts that must be followed identically for every patient. The key, he emphasized, is flexibility paired with consistency (Whitehouse & Stukus, 2026).

Dr. Stukus is a board-certified pediatric allergist, Professor of Clinical Pediatrics, and Director of the Food Allergy Treatment Center at Nationwide Children's Hospital. He is also the 2025-2026 President-Elect of the American College of Allergy, Asthma and Immunology and a nationally recognized leader in the field of allergy and immunology. He emphasized that treatment must be shaped around the patient and family, not the other way around. Sports schedules, family arrangements, work demands, travel, other medical needs, picky eating, and an infinite number of other factors influence how each patient's immunotherapy will proceed.

Confirming the Diagnosis

One of the most important steps before OIT is ensuring that the patient is truly allergic to the food in question. Dr. Stukus emphasized the dangers of over-testing. Panel testing without a clear clinical history frequently leads to false positives and unnecessary dietary restrictions.

Testing alone should never create a diagnosis. Allergy tests should be used to support a diagnosis that is already suggested by a clinical history and a reproducible reaction. If someone is eating a food regularly without symptoms, they are not allergic to it. Undoing an incorrect diagnosis can require food challenges and repeat testing before immunotherapy starts to avoid a lengthy treatment process for a food the patient is not truly allergic to. Clarifying which foods are truly allergens can reduce the emotional and logistical burden dramatically (Whitehouse & Stukus, 2026).

The Role of Food Challenges

Food challenges are often a part of this diagnostic clarification process, and are also often the most feared part of preparation. Dr. Stukus countered that they can also be among the most empowering. At centers like the Food Allergy Treatment Center at Nationwide Children's Hospital, Dr. Stukus and his team frequently use what they call a threshold challenge. Small doses of an allergen are given and gradually increased under close observation to determine how much the patient can tolerate before symptoms begin.

Contrary to common fears, Dr. Stukus emphasized that reactions rarely move rapidly from zero to severe. More often, the first signs are subtle changes like a few hives, a shift in behavior from playful to withdrawn, or mild stomach discomfort. These early signs provide valuable information, and allow for treatment to be administered calmly if needed. Parents are guided through the process and, if needed, administer epinephrine themselves under supervision so they can experience what it feels like in a controlled setting (Whitehouse & Stukus, 2026). Dr. Stukus' experience is consistent with research showing that epinephrine administration in a supervised setting reduces fear rather than amplifies it (Theodorakakis et al., 2024). The unknown becomes familiar, and the imagined catastrophe becomes a manageable medical event.

Knowing What to Expect

Dr. Stukus pointed out that many patients who are not having an allergic reaction might notice that their throat feels strange the first time they intentionally eat a food they have avoided for years. Butterflies in the stomach, thick saliva, and a tight sensation are common anxiety responses that present as very real physical symptoms. These sensations are the brain's alarm system reacting to something it knows is potentially dangerous, not necessarily allergic reactions.

Parents are coached to avoid repetitive or leading questioning such as "Do you feel okay?" Dr. Stukus' experience is that distraction and calm presence are the best ways to regulate the moment. It is also critical to address distorted risk perceptions before beginning OIT. Correcting exaggerated risk perceptions reduces the likelihood that every sneeze during OIT will be interpreted as disaster.

Extremely high anxiety does not automatically disqualify a family from OIT, but an open conversation about it is usually helpful. The hope, and the common outcome, is that treatment reduces anxiety in the long term by increasing tolerance and safety (Whitehouse & Stukus, 2026).

Practical Logistics

Preparation also includes a clear look at daily life. Doses are typically given with a full stomach, followed by a rest period during which vigorous exercise is avoided. That does not mean that the patient must sit still for two hours. It means no intense physical exertion.

Schedules, custody arrangements, travel plans, sports practices, babysitters, and school activities all need careful consideration. In some cases, doses can be split between morning and evening to make larger volumes more manageable. The principles of OIT rely on consistent exposure over time, not perfection.

Missed doses happen, and most patients can resume after short interruptions without significant issues. These decisions are individualized and guided by the treating allergist.

Dr. Stukus shared that a common reason he has seen families discontinue OIT is taste fatigue. Eating the same food daily that the patient dislikes can become exhausting. Creative strategies such as varying delivery of the food, using savory options instead of sweet ones, and baking carefully portioned items can help. Still, if the patient cannot bring themselves to eat it regularly, forcing it may create more harm than benefit. Some families choose to remain at a lower maintenance dose and others pause and revisit treatment later (Whitehouse & Stukus, 2026).

Research shows that gastrointestinal side effects are another leading reason patients and families discontinue OIT. Other common factors are allergic reactions with up-dosing, anaphylaxis, eosinophilic esophagitis (EoE), difficulty with dose administration, treatment burden, anxiety about reactions, and lifestyle challenges (Plessis et al., 2024). There is no failure in stopping treatment or maintaining a smaller dose than initially planned. The experience itself provides learning and exposure that may reduce fear moving forward.

Flexibility Within the Routine

Research trials over time have provided critical data about safety and dosing ranges. They do not dictate a single correct pathway. Dr. Stukus emphasized that protocols can be individualized. The goal is not to achieve an arbitrarily high daily dose of the allergen (Whitehouse & Stukus, 2026). Recent research demonstrates that even low maintenance doses can provide meaningful protection against accidental exposures (Sato et al., 2025).

Families should feel empowered to ask what level of protection a given maintenance dose provides and what tradeoffs are involved. Thoughtful treatment planning is collaborative. In Dr. Stukus' experience, the most important marker of success is comfort with the decision. Preparing well medically and mentally does not eliminate uncertainty, but it replaces catastrophic imagination with lived experience, informed choice, and realistic expectations (Whitehouse & Stukus, 2026).

Preparing My Son for OIT

By the time we were ready to pursue OIT, I had spent years navigating the unpredictable and often frightening world of food allergies. That experience shaped not only how I approached treatment for my son, but also how I prepared myself as a parent. Preparation is multidimensional: emotional, logistical, financial, and relational. Acknowledging each of these areas can make a significant difference in the experience and outcomes of immunotherapy.

Emotional Preparation

Perhaps the most challenging aspect of preparing for treatment is the emotional work. As a parent, I carried a mix of hope, fear, and exhaustion. I worried constantly about reactions, the process itself, and whether we could manage it all without letting anxiety take over. At the same time, I needed to maintain calm in front of my children, even when inside I was tense and fearful.

Through this journey, I learned that emotional preparation is about more than "staying calm." It requires acknowledging your own feelings, noticing the ways your body responds to stress, and developing strategies to regulate your nervous system. This includes recognizing the anxiety that arises when talking to doctors, reading about treatments, or imagining your child taking their first doses. Naming these feelings, allowing yourself to feel them, and having a plan to manage them can help you approach treatment in a grounded and attuned way.

My son's immediate comfort with our doctor seemed to calm his uneasiness about the process. He liked the idea of teaching his immune system that peanuts were food, not poison. Since we did not typically drink it at home, the fact that his doses would be flavored with grape Kool-Aid felt novel and exciting to him. At the office, we showed him how the dose would be an invisible amount of peanut mixed into the drink, explaining that his body would slowly learn not to react to it.

Physical Preparation

Scheduling appointments, traveling to clinics, arranging childcare for my younger children, structuring our days around daily doses at home, enforcing the rest period, and monitoring for reactions required stamina and organization. We would be making the 8-hour round-trip adventure every two weeks, and that meant adjusting our entire work schedules and daily routine. Looking back, I can see that it was pure hope motivating me through the work it took to make these arrangements and stick to that routine for years. (It took us longer than typical to move through my son's multiple allergens while navigating his high sensitivity and reactivity.)

I also feel fortunate that my son did great with car travel. He loved to read in the car, and we also picked out podcasts that we would listen to together. We made lists of comfort items that would feel supportive to him, meals and snacks to pack that he would enjoy, and things to do to keep busy during the long wait at the clinic. The food routine stuck throughout the experience, with my son happily eating his cold homemade pizza every two weeks in the car just before arriving to ensure he had a full stomach for his updose. His choice of entertainment shifted over time, and was easy to keep fresh to make his time more enjoyable for him and calm for me.

Financial Preparation

Before starting, I sat down and made lists, estimated the frequency of visits, and considered both direct and indirect costs. I also looked carefully at the decrease in my work that would be required, and the long term financial impact of that change. Thinking ahead allowed me to plan, rather than be blindsided, and helped me reduce stress once the treatment began. While cost is a practical concern, the emotional and relational investments are just as significant. At this point, I'd have given anything to increase my sensitive son's safety.

Relational Preparation and Trusting Your Providers

One of the most important lessons from my early experiences was the need for a trusting partnership with healthcare providers. After our past discouraging experiences, finding a practice that was willing to collaborate, listen, and treat my knowledge and experiences as assets completely shifted how I experienced the process. A provider that took the time to explain options, answer questions, and engage me in shared decision-making helped my nervous system relax and my confidence grow so that I was better able to support my child. I remember consciously looking at the doctor's warm face during an appointment and telling myself silently, "You just have to trust him." Luckily, that felt possible based on our experiences with him.

Preparation also extended to my husband and my mother, who would be helping us with childcare. Consistent communication, shared expectations, and understanding everyone's role helped to reduce confusion, prevent misunderstandings, and ensured that our son was always supported. My husband happily made the homemade pizza the night before each appointment, and packed the food while I fed the children and spent time with the younger kids before leaving.

The two little brothers even found a place in the bi-weekly routine. Every appointment, they ensured that we arrived home to a homemade sign waiting on the door celebrating that week's achievement. At first they were scribbles with their Dad's handwriting dictating their words of encouragement. Over the years they evolved into hilarious cartoons, usually some variation of my son wrestling or beating up a nut. We lined our kitchen walls with them, and didn't take them down until well after he had reached maintenance. Those small routines of support and connection became some of the most meaningful memories of our OIT days.

Bringing It All Together
Preparing for immunotherapy was not simply a checklist of appointments and dosages. It was an ongoing process of building confidence, developing coping strategies and routines, and creating systems of support. Emotional regulation, physical organization, financial planning, and relational alignment all worked together to help everyone in the family navigate the challenges and opportunities of treatment. Investing some extra energy in preparation up front gave us all greater clarity, resilience, and a sense of agency.

Additional Resource
Hope for Henry's resource hub offers helpful guides for preparing children for common medical procedures, including allergy skin testing and blood draws. Their resource hub includes child-friendly explanations and practical strategies to help families approach these experiences with more confidence and less fear.

Skin Testing: https://hub.hopeforhenry.org/resources/allergytesting/
Blood Testing: https://hub.hopeforhenry.org/procedure/blood-test/

Preparing for Treatment – Mapping Your Readiness

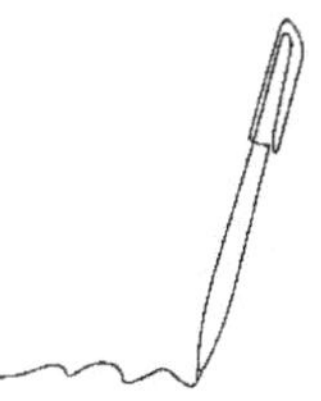

Immunotherapy is a journey that involves more than just medical appointments and doses. Being prepared emotionally, physically, financially, and relationally helps you and your child feel more confident, supported, and able to navigate challenges. Use this page to explore each area, reflect on what you need, and make a plan.

Emotional Preparation

What emotions come up when you think about doses, potential reactions, or preparing for/attending appointments?

- How do I feel about the treatment process?
- What worries or fears come up for me? What worries or fears has my child voiced?
- What strategies help each of us regulate stress?
- What support or resources might help us feel more confident?

____

____

____

____

____

Physical Preparation

Consider what practical steps you'll need to take for treatment.

- What routines or schedules will need to change?
- Who can help with childcare, preparation, transportation, or supervision during doses?
- How will we all maintain wellness (sleep, nutrition, exercise)?

____

____

____

____

____

Financial Preparation

Treatment often involves direct and indirect costs. Use this section to plan for your estimated costs. Revisit the previous workbook page on financial considerations in Chapter 4 if helpful.

- Appointment costs, co-pays, or medications
- Specialized foods, equipment, or home supplies
- Travel, parking, or lodging if applicable
- Time off work or adjustments to schedules

Relational Preparation

Consider how to prepare partners, family, friends, co-workers, school staff, and coparents.

- Who else needs to be informed about the treatment plan?
- How will I communicate expectations and routines?
- How can we ensure consistency across households if needed?
- How can we support each other emotionally during this process?

Trusting Your Providers

Your relationship with your medical team can profoundly impact your experience.

- Do I feel comfortable asking questions and sharing my observations?
- Do I feel listened to and respected as a partner in care?
- Are there concerns I need to address or clarify before treatment begins?

Final Reflection:

- What feels most manageable?
- What feels most challenging?
- What is one step I can take to increase my readiness?

My Goals for Treatment

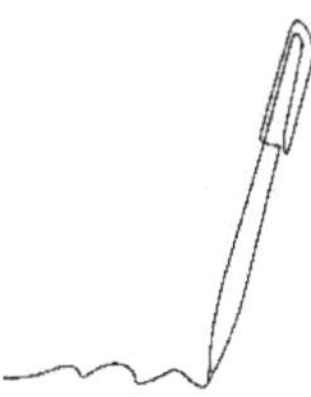

This exercise helps you move from abstract hopes into clear, meaningful direction. Return to this throughout the process to stay motivated or re-evaluate your progress. Consider putting a visual reminder somewhere to inspire you.

What Am I Hoping to Change?

Right now, what feels most limiting or difficult?

____

____

What Do I Want More Of?

Safety / medical:

____

____

Daily life / routines:

____

____

Social experiences:

____

____

Emotional experience:

____

____

Holding Flexibility

This process may not unfold exactly as expected.

What would it look like to stay committed to your direction, even if the path changes?

____

____

Closing Reflection

You may not control every outcome, but you can stay connected to the direction you've chosen.

My Goals for Treatment

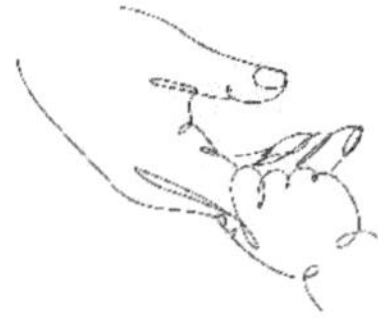 Before beginning treatment, get clear on something that will motivate your child to complete the treatment. They can be anything from huge things like eating a whole serving of their allergen to things that seem small to you as a parent.
Your child can write, draw, or use stickers, or ask you to record their answers.

What Do You Hope For?

☐ Eating a certain food

☐ Going certain places without worry

☐ Eating with friends

☐ Trying new restaurants

☐ Feeling less:

Other:

What I hope for the most is:

What would it look and feel like for that to happen?

When Coping Takes the Lead

 There is something I have come to understand about myself only in hindsight, and it took years of distance and gentleness to see it clearly. Most of the time, I am a warm, affectionate, emotionally present mother. I am physically close, expressive, and attuned. That is how I know myself, and that is how my children know me.

Under acute stress related to my son's allergies, however, a different version of me takes the lead. When the stakes feel high and the threat feels real, my system shifts into competence mode. I become focused, organized, and task-oriented. I work hard to remain neutral on the outside, to not show fear, to not unravel. My attention goes to logistics, problem solving, phone calls, planning, and preparing for what might be coming next. In those moments, efficiency replaces softness, not because I do not care, but because my nervous system has decided that action is what will keep everyone safe.

Looking back, I can see how this played out during medical emergencies. I was doing everything that needed to be done. But there are moments I wish I had held him longer, offered more comfort, or allowed myself to be softer alongside being capable. I can see now that I could have done both. At the time, that option was not easily available to me. This pattern was a nervous system response, not a failure of love or attunement.

When we are under threat, especially when our child's safety is involved, our nervous system prioritizes survival. For some people, that looks like heightened emotion or panic. For others, it looks like shutting down feelings in order to function. Neither response is chosen consciously. They are adaptive strategies shaped by our wiring, our experiences, and what our system has learned works.

What I have learned is that how we show up in everyday life is not always how we show up in crisis. The version of you that exists under stress may surprise you, and that does not mean it is more "true" than the rest of you. It means your nervous system is doing its best to protect what matters most.

I share this not to judge my past self, but to offer compassion to the parts of me that stepped in when things felt overwhelming. This section of the book is an invitation to do the same for yourself: to notice your own patterns under stress without labeling them as wrong, and to understand that coping styles shift in emergencies. Awareness, not self criticism, is what allows new options to emerge over time.

Understanding Your Coping Style Under Stress

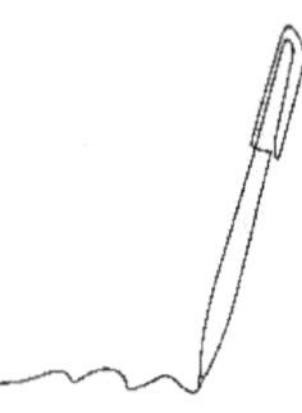

This page is designed to help you notice how your nervous system responds during high stress situations. There are no right or wrong answers. The goal is to increase awareness of how our nervous systems naturally respond, not to create guilt or shame.

How I Show Up Most of the Time

Take a moment to describe how you typically handle tasks for yourself or relate to your child when things feel relatively calm.

Words that describe me most days:
(example: affectionate, playful, patient, attentive)

____

____

How I usually seek comfort for myself, and how I try to provide it to others:
(physical closeness, talking things through, humor, reassurance)

____

____

How I Show Up Under Stress or In Emergencies

Now think about moments when safety felt uncertain or when fear was high.

What I tend to focus on first:

☐ Tasks and logistics

☐ Information and details

☐ Monitoring symptoms

☐ Emotional reassurance

☐ Other: ____

What happens to my emotions in those moments:

☐ I feel everything intensely

☐ I feel numb or detached

☐ I push feelings aside to function

☐ It varies depending on the situation

☐ Other: ____

Changes I notice in my body or behavior:
(tightness, urgency, silence, hyperfocus, restlessness)

____

____

Naming the Protective Role of This Pattern

Instead of asking, "What's wrong with this response?" try asking:

What might my nervous system be trying to accomplish or protect in those moments?

____

____

In what ways has this response helped me or my child?

____

____

Holding Compassion and Curiosity Together

You are not being asked to change anything here. Just notice.

Something I can offer myself compassion for in these moments:

____

____

One gentle question or curiosity I can observe:
(examples: What would support look like for me in moments like this?
What need am I trying to meet?)

____

____

Reminder

Most of us have responses that are beyond our awareness during emergencies, and these are usually protective or caring in some way even if they are something we would like to change. Awareness is the first step toward choice, and choice only becomes available when the nervous system feels safe enough to notice.

Understanding Your Child's Reactions and Patterns

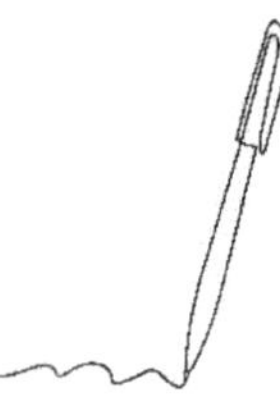

This worksheet helps parents notice how their child responds under stress, fear, or after a medical event. It is meant to help you observe and learn, *not as questions that you should pose to your child*. Understanding your child's patterns allows for more targeted support and helps you co-regulate effectively.

Observe and Describe

How does my child usually react during a stressful or medical situation?

☐ Withdraws or becomes quiet

☐ Gets irritable or angry

☐ Attempts to distract themselves

☐ Cries or expresses fear

☐ Clings for reassurance

☐ Other: ______________________________

What physical signs do I notice in my child when stressed?
(racing heart, fidgeting, flushed skin, holding stomach, shallow breathing, loss of appetite, etc.)

____

____

How does my child recover once the immediate stressor has passed?

☐ Quickly returns to baseline

☐ Needs extra comfort or play

☐ Gets emotional (angry, sad, energetic, silly)

☐ Needs time alone

☐ Seeks connection and conversation

☐ Other: ______________________________

Understanding Triggers

What tends to trigger the strongest reactions in my child?
(specific medical procedures, waiting rooms, blood draws, changes in routine, new environments)

____

____

What helps them calm down most quickly?
(touch, breathing exercises, favorite toy, conversation, storytelling)

____

____

Reflection

How does my own stress influence my child's reaction? (Think of specific examples if possible)

____

____

Co-Regulation and Repair After Medical Events

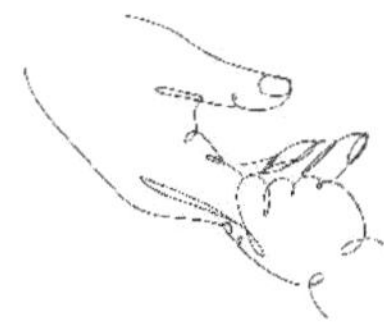 These activities help parents guide children through emotional regulation and processing after medical experiences and strengthen the parent-child connection.

Recognize and Label Emotions

Share something you observed, the emotion that it suggested, and validate it. Don't argue with your child if they deny that feeling or describe their emotions differently.

- o Ex. "You balled up your fists and held your mouth closed tight. It seemed like you felt afraid of the dose. This is all a lot to understand and get used to.
- o For children who aren't as verbally expressive, use a feelings chart or the emojis on a phone or tablet to let your child point to or color the emotions they felt.

Co-Regulate Together

Your nervous system cues your child's. Think of lending them your calm, regulated energy to help them feel safer and calmer.

Under 5:

- Deep belly breathing (the parent breathing deeply and slowly helps the child do so, too)
- Rocking, swaying, or dancing together
- Cuddling with you and a favorite stuffed animal/comfort item
- Hands on activities like drawing, coloring, painting, modeling clay, sand, water beads

Ages 5–9:

- Guided breathing (pretend you're blowing up a balloon or blowing out birthday candles)
- Coloring or drawing about the experience
- Letting the child tell the story in a homemade book or puppet show with favorite toys
- A walk outside, stomping up stairs, wrapping up in a blanket

Ages 10 and up:

- Meditation or mindfulness activity together
- Expressing feelings together through conversation, journaling, art, or music
- Movement: going for a walk, partner yoga or stretches, playing a sport
- Physical comfort (most big kids and adults are soothed by hugs, backrubs, hand-holding, etc.)

Chapter 6:
Strengthening Routines and Connections

Strengthening Routines Before Immunotherapy

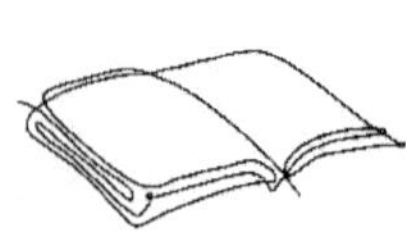

Immunotherapy doesn't start on the first dosing day. Long before clinic visits, measuring, and vigilance, individuals and families are anticipating how life will change. It is natural to focus on logistics, risks, and medical readiness, but equally important to prepare the individual and family system to navigate uncertainty, repetition, and stress. One of the most effective ways to build this capacity is through establishing consistent, predictable routines before treatment begins.

Why Routines Matter in Times of Medical Stress

Research consistently shows that routines and rituals support emotional wellbeing for both children and adults. They create predictability, reinforce connection, and provide a sense of safety during uncertain times (Fiese et al., 2002; Spagnola & Fiese, 2007). Daily routines reduce cognitive and emotional load by signaling what comes next, supporting nervous system regulation and lowering baseline stress, which is critical when navigating chronic medical care (Fiese & Everhart, 2006).

Family rituals also strengthen emotional security and parent–child connection in households managing chronic conditions. Shared, repeated moments help children feel held within something steady, even when other parts of life feel unpredictable. Over time, these rituals contribute to resilience, offering a reliable place to return to regardless of daily disruptions (Crespo et al., 2013).

Routines as a Protective Factor in Medical Treatment

In households managing chronic illness, consistent routines act as a protective factor. They are linked to better emotional adjustment, improved adherence to medical care, and stronger family cohesion (Fiese & Everhart, 2006). Immunotherapy introduces new stressors, and practicing any new routines before treatment helps to build a foundation of regulation and connection that treatment can rest on, rather than compete with.

Preparing for Immunotherapy Through Routine

Routines provide emotional containment during anticipatory stress, create predictable touchpoints of connection, provide consistency, and reduce decision fatigue (Fiese & Everhart, 2006). Routines help to practice familiarity with repeated steps and signals, laying a foundation for the structured, daily nature of OIT.

Effective routines are consistent, meaningful, and manageable. They don't need to be rigid, elaborate, or time-consuming. The goal is to create moments of steadiness that signal safety to the nervous system, helping the family feel grounded even during uncertainty (Fiese et al., 2002). Consider what will need to happen daily, and begin implementing it before treatment begins.

Examples of Immunotherapy Routines

- *Medical prep practice:* Practicing routines like organizing the dosing area, washing hands, or practicing taking a small "practice" dose of a safe food can lay the foundation and structure and steps of immunotherapy. Children can even practice taking a pretend "dose" of water or juice from a syringe.

- *Meals before dosing:* Choose the time and place that dosing will take place and practice it. It can be helpful to think ahead to meals and snacks that the patient consistently enjoys to ensure that they will have enough to eat before dosing.

- *Calm activities:* Quiet play or activities support the rest time required after dosing. Legos, puzzles, card games, board games, and art activities work well. Have a selection on hand to prevent boredom, and do these with children to increase their interest and co-regulation.

- *Visual schedules or charts:* Using a calendar or chart to track routines, daily doses, appointments, and overall progress helps to anticipate what comes next and celebrate small successes. (This is motivating for big kids and adults, too, not just little ones!)

Practicing these routines before treatment begins builds a foundation of familiarity, connection, and regulation that immunotherapy can build upon, rather than compete with. In uncertain times, predictability is a form of safety and connection.

Routines That Support Regulation and Connection

 This page offers ideas for simple, meaningful family routines that support emotional regulation and connection before and during immunotherapy. These routines are meant to be sustainable, adaptable, and grounded in real family life. Use this page for inspiration. You do not need to do all or many of these. One or two consistent routines can make a meaningful difference.

Early Childhood (Under 5)

Young children benefit most from routines that are sensory based, predictable, and relational.

- A short bedtime rhythm that happens in the same order each night (bath, book, song)
- A consistent phrase or gesture used before transitions
- A daily cuddle or other moment of affection at the same time/place each day
- Singing the same song during car rides or before stressful events
- A shared joke, handshake, or symbolic gesture before separation

Elementary Age (approximately ages 5 to 10)

Children in this stage benefit from routines that combine predictability with voice and participation.

- A weekly family meal where everyone shares one win or goal for the week
- A short walk together after dinner on certain nights
- A consistent check-in before school or bedtime
- A weekly game night or puzzle night
- Creating a simple tradition before appointments (same snack, same music)

Tweens and Teens (approximately ages 11 and up)

Adolescents often resist routines that feel imposed, but benefit from rituals that respect autonomy while maintaining connection.

- A regular shared meal without phones
- A predictable weekly check in that allows them to express wants/needs
- A shared activity that does not require conversation (walking, driving, watching a show)
- A consistent way of reconnecting after hard days
- A routine around appointments that includes choice and control

Updose Appointment Day Routine

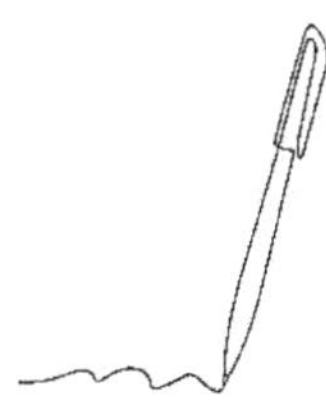

This page will help you create a predictable, supportive routine for clinic updose days, to reduce stress and to help you feel safe and prepared. This will likely change over time for many reasons, so repeat the activity if it becomes clear that you need to adjust. (If your child is the patient, get their input where helpful but plan what you can without them.)

Tip: Designate a bag for appointment days and use it each time. Pack the night before and keep it in the same place before appointments. Consider letting kids pack their own small bag using the activity on the next page.

Before the Appointment

☐ Appointment time: ____

☐ Pre-dose meal/snack: ____

☐ Pre-appointment meds/doses ____

☐ Who is attending: ____

☐ Childcare for siblings (if needed) ____

☐ Explain what to expect today ____

☐ Gas in vehicle to eliminate unnecessary stops on the way home (if driving)

During the Appointment

☐ Make note of dose/changes ____

☐ Plan for observation period ____

☐ Comfort strategies for waiting ____

After the Appointment

☐ Easy, low-effort meal plan for later ____

☐ Quiet activities ready at home ____

☐ Small joy/comfort/celebration ____

To Pack:

Essentials for Dosing & Safety

☐ Prescribed emergency medications (epinephrine devices)

☐ Antihistamine, inhaler, and any other medications recommended by your allergist

☐ Emergency Action Plan (always keep a paper copy with your epinephrine)

☐ Insurance card / ID

☐ List of questions for the allergist

☐ Notes from previous doses

☐ Other ____

Food & Drink (for patient and any caregivers joining them)

☐ Foods for before or after dosing

☐ Foods for the actual dose (the allergen being dosed; pre-measured if necessary)

☐ Food needed to mix the dose with (if applicable; applesauce, pudding, etc.)

☐ Preferred snacks (familiar, easy-to-eat options)

☐ Drinks (water, electrolyte drink, etc.)

☐ Other ____

Comfort & Regulation

☐ Favorite comfort item (stuffed animal, blanket, etc.)

☐ Headphones or calming music

☐ Tablet/phone + charger

☐ Books, puzzles, activity/sticker books, card games, quiet activities

☐ Sensory tools like fidgets for tactile input or oral motor stimulation (gum, mints, chewelry)

☐ Visual calming items (photo album, kaleidoscope, hourglass timer, glitter jar)

☐ Affirmation cards or coping skills cards

☐ Layers of clothing for comfort in office heat/air conditioning

☐ Other ____

Practical Items

☐ Change of clothes (in case of spills, reactions, car sickness, etc.)

☐ Tissues/wipes

☐ Small trash bags, zip-top bags, emesis bags (in case of vomiting) for messes

☐ Wipes (for hands and to clean surfaces)

☐ Creams (e.g., for skin irritation)

☐ Other ____

Appointment Prep Scavenger Hunt

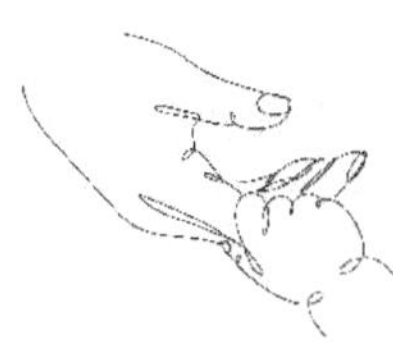 Let's make getting ready for your appointment a game! This scavenger hunt will help you find the things that will keep you comfortable, calm, and entertained during your appointment. (Parents, it is recommended to do this 2-3 days before the appointment, not the night before. Choose a special bag that will only be used for appointments.)

As you find each item, check it off, add a sticker or draw it in your bag below!

Can you find something…

☐ Comfortable to wear

☐ That makes you feel cozy (like a favorite sweatshirt, blanket, or soft item)

☐ That helps you pass the time (book, game, puzzle, or activity)

☐ That lets you listen to something (headphones, music, audiobook)

☐ That makes you smile or laugh

☐ That helps you feel calm when you're nervous

☐ That you really enjoy using or playing with

☐ That you can use quietly while waiting

☐ That feels like a little piece of home

☐ To show your medical team or waiting room friends

☐ That makes you feel proud or confident

Draw or write your favorite thing you chose for this appointment

My Dosing Buddy

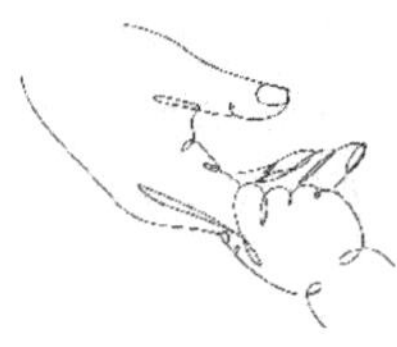 Sometimes it helps to have something or someone familiar with you during new or challenging experiences. You are going to choose a buddy who will stay with you throughout your treatment journey. Invite children to draw or write their answers, or to have you record their responses for them.

Choose A Buddy and Draw Them Here

Your buddy can be: a stuffed animal, a favorite character, a special object that feels special to you

What did you choose?

Get to Know Your Buddy

What kind of buddy will they be?

What will make them a good helper?

Your Buddy's Job

What would you like your buddy to do on appointment days and during dosing?

☐ sit with you during appointments   ☐ practice doses with you

☐ listen when you talk about how things feel   ☐ remind you that you're not alone

What else would you like your buddy to help with?

Coping Skills Sandwich

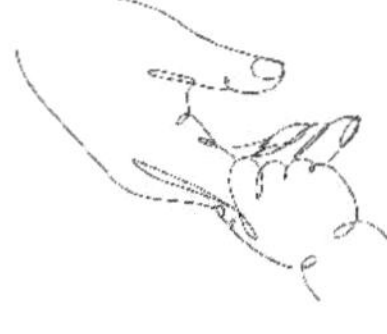 When emotions feel big, it helps to have a plan, especially a plan that was created and practiced before those big feelings flared. This activity helps children create their own "coping skills sandwich," a simple way to remember what helps them feel safe, supported, and prepared.

This activity builds two things at the same time:

Coping Skills (What helps my body and feelings settle?)
Allergy Safety (What foods are safe for me?)

Prepping Ingredients

Cut out and color the sandwich pieces. Each ingredient represents a different kind of support. Encourage your child to choose what "ingredients" belong in their coping sandwich.

Holding It All Together

No matter what ingredients you put inside your sandwich, it has something on the outside to hold everything together. It might be bread, pita, a tortilla, or even a lettuce wrap. Whatever it is, it connects all the ingredients and makes it what it is: a sandwich.

Whatever you choose to hold your sandwich together represents connection, the first and last step of coping and making a sandwich. Always start by identifying who helps you feel safe and supported, and what makes you feel close to them. This might be: parents, grandparents, aunts and uncles, siblings, teachers, friends, school staff, therapists, or other trusted people in your life.

Choosing Safe Ingredients

Add any sandwich ingredients you like that are safe for you while discussing things that help you feel safe and calm. Draw and add any ingredients of your own that aren't shown here!

Practice identifying allergens and safe alternatives as ingredients are selected. Then practice a coping skill for each topping as you choose it. (See the "menu" on the next page for ideas.)

Stack & Enjoy

Pile your sandwich high with as many ingredients as you like and (pretend to) enjoy!

SANDWICH MENU

BREAD / WRAP = CONNECTION
(Support from someone trusted and safe)

Ask for a hug	Hold someone's hand	Sit next to them
Text or call a parent	Tell the teacher or nurse	Ask for help
Stay close to them	Tell them/listen to a joke	Code word/handshake

SANDWICH MEAT / PROTEIN = RELAXATION
(Ways to calm the body and mind)

Deep breathing	Blow a pinwheel	Blow bubbles
Listen to calming sounds	Blow out pretend birthday candles	Squeeze pillow/stuffie

CHEESE = PHYSICAL / SENSORY REGULATION
(Using body energy to reduce tension)

Fidget toys	Dancing	Running
Jumping	Playing with clay or slime	Squeezing a stress ball
Swinging	Stomping up stairs	Push on a wall

VEGGIES = COGNITIVE / THINKING SKILLS
(Changing unhelpful thoughts)

Positive self-talk like:	"I can do hard things"	"This feeling will pass"
Naming emotions	Thinking of a favorite memory	Counting slowly

CONDIMENTS = REDIRECTION
(Activities that help shift focus somewhere else)

Drawing	Listening to music	Reading a book
Playing a game	Watching something funny	Telling jokes
Coloring	Singing	Doing a puzzle

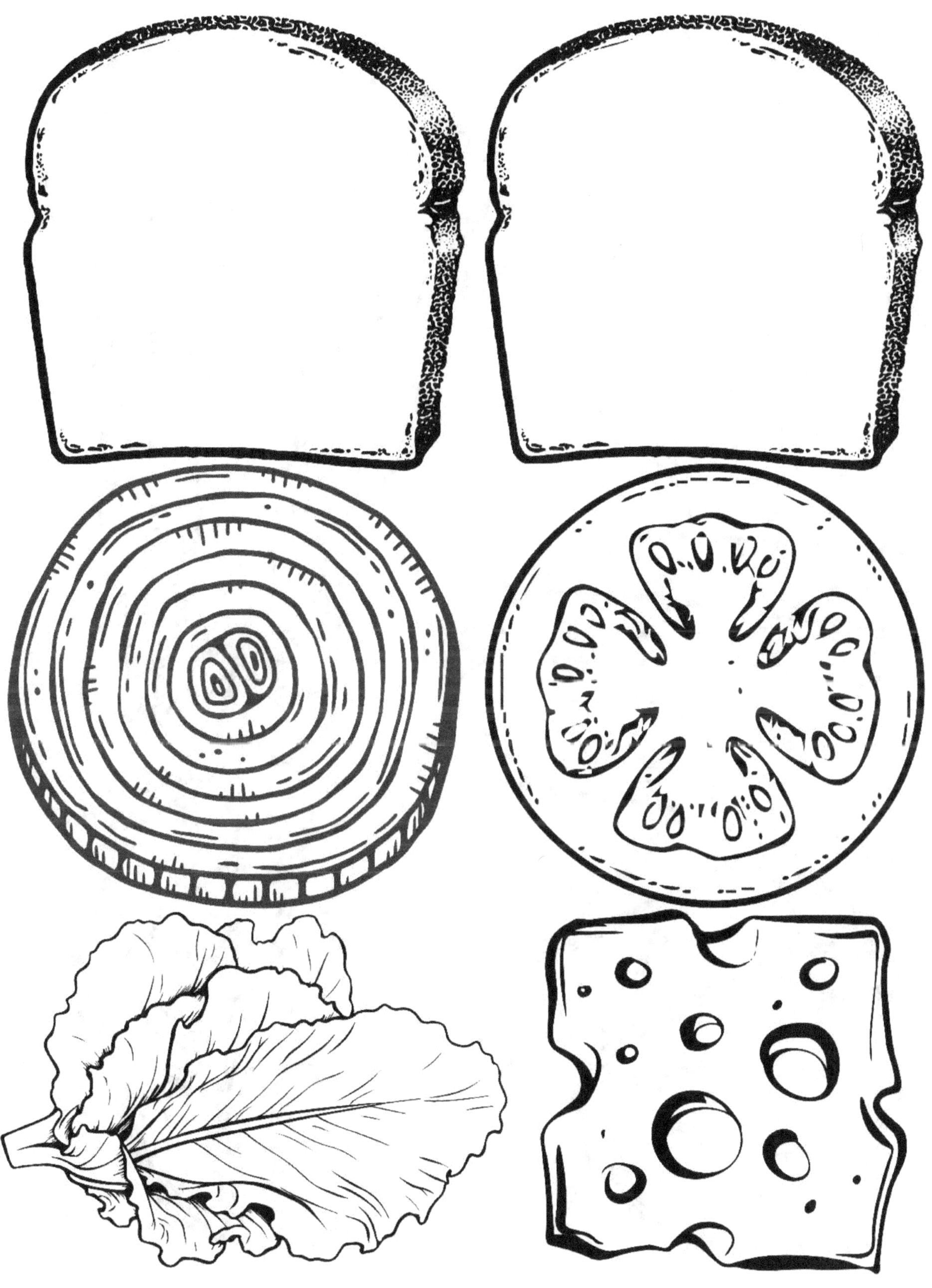

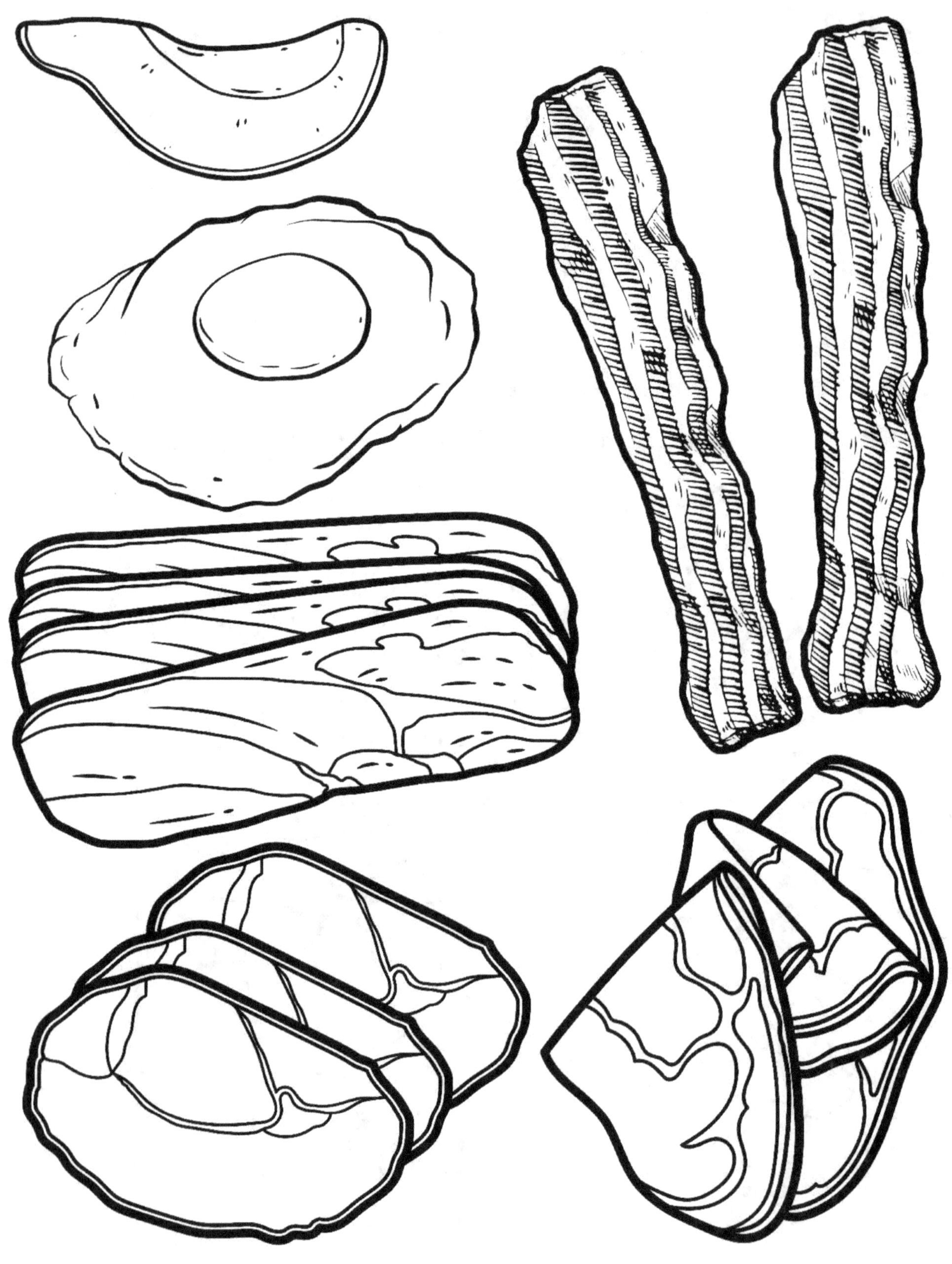

S
P

Chapter 7:
Understanding Fear in Medical Moments

Using Epinephrine Without Hesitation

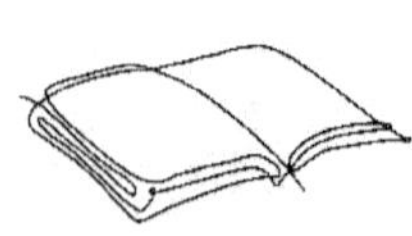 When and whether to use epinephrine is one of the most common stressors reported by patients and parents. Fear, conflicting messages, past negative experiences of shame, and the desire to avoid making the "wrong" call all contribute to this. This becomes even more complicated when beginning immunotherapy, because your doctor might give you slightly different instructions for epinephrine use after dosing.

Parents are told epinephrine is lifesaving, yet many have experienced mixed messaging about when to use it. Some have been criticized by emergency personnel after symptoms resolved. Others worry about hurting themselves or their child, triggering an emergency room visit, being judged for "overreacting," or using their expensive medicine unnecessarily.

Dr. Farah Khan is a board-certified allergist/immunologist and pediatrician at Nationwide Children's Hospital, where she specializes in caring for children with allergic conditions and complex immune disorders. She is also a widely recognized voice in allergy education, sharing evidence-based information with a large online audience through her social media platform @farah.khan.md. One of the things she is known for is challenging epinephrine fear and hesitation, and her phrase "Use the dang epi" has resonated with thousands of patients and parents. On episode 67 of the *Don't Feed the Fear* podcast, Dr. Khan noted that her personal style may be direct, but the message behind it is grounded in decades of allergy research and clinical experience (Whitehouse & Khan, 2026).

The Most Common Epinephrine Myths

One of the most persistent misconceptions is that epinephrine should only be used when someone is struggling to breathe. In reality, waiting for breathing difficulty is waiting far too long because other allergic reaction symptoms may already be present. Dr. Khan emphasized that involvement of more than one body system is enough reason to use epinephrine. An allergy action plan outlining these body systems and associated symptoms should be discussed with your own provider.

Another common belief is that using epinephrine automatically requires calling 911 or going to the emergency room. While emergency care is sometimes necessary, evolving guidelines and post-pandemic practices recognize that if symptoms resolve and the individual is stable, patients may be able to monitor safely at home. Fear of an ER visit should never be the reason epinephrine is withheld, and patients should discuss a plan for this with their own doctors when reviewing their allergy action plans.

Perhaps the most emotionally charged myth is the fear of "being wrong." Many worry about using epinephrine when it turns out the reaction would not have progressed. The medical reality is simple and reassuring: epinephrine is safe. The body produces it naturally. If it is given and turns out not to have been strictly necessary, it does not cause harm. Not using it when it is needed is where the danger lies (Whitehouse & Khan, 2026).

Choosing an Epinephrine Device

Today, families have more epinephrine options than ever before. Traditional auto injectors, voice guided devices, intranasal epinephrine, and emerging sublingual options all contain the same medication. The only difference is in the delivery system.

Side effects exist with all medications. Nasal epinephrine may sting or burn. Injectors may cause soreness or bruising. These potential trade-offs should be discussed openly with your allergist so you can make informed decisions without fear or pressure (Whitehouse & Khan, 2026).

What Matters Most

Epinephrine is not a last resort. It is the first line treatment for anaphylaxis. Using it promptly can prevent escalation, reduce the need for intensive emergency care, and save lives. If you have any uncertainty about your epinephrine device or when to use it in everyday life or in the context of immunotherapy, it is important to have a conversation with your doctor for clarity and confidence in your ability to respond to an emergency. Dr. Khan emphasized one guiding principle above all others: the best epinephrine is the one you will carry and use (Whitehouse & Khan, 2026).

Additional Reading

For further reading that goes into more depth about general medical anxiety and trauma, *Afraid of the Doctor: Every Parent's Guide to Preventing and Managing Medical Trauma* by Megan Marsac and Melissa Hogan is a highly recommended resource.

Epinephrine Fear and Hesitation

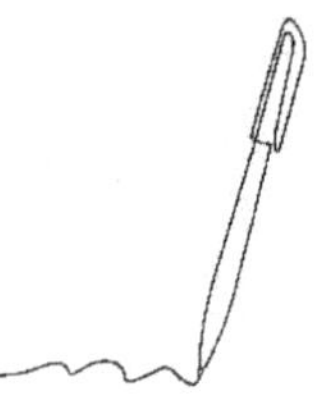

Epinephrine hesitation can be a combination of many factors including not knowing what to do or when to do it, fear, past experiences or trauma, mixed messaging, guilt, shame, financial strain, and the universal urge to avoid doing the "wrong" thing. This page helps you gently map what comes up for you so those fears can be named, understood, and worked with rather than ignored or shamed.

There are no right or wrong answers. Awareness comes first. Confidence grows from there.

Identify Your Immediate Thoughts

When you imagine a moment where epinephrine might be needed, what thoughts come up first?

☐ What if I'm overreacting? ☐ What if it hurts?

☐ What if I use it and it turns out I didn't need it? ☐ What if we have to go to the ER?

☐ What if I waste this expensive medication? ☐ What if I panic and freeze?

Let your thoughts flow and write anything else that comes to mind:

____

____

____

____

Notice the Underlying Fear

Often, the surface thought is not the core fear. Ask yourself what feels threatening underneath.

☐ Fear of causing harm ☐ Fear of being judged

☐ Fear of being wrong or making a mistake ☐ Fear of the intensity of the experience

☐ Fear of emergency care ☐ Fear of past scary experience(s)

☐ Fear that using epi means there was real danger ☐ Fear of losing control

☐ Fear rooted in a previous reaction or emergency ☐ Fear of needles or pain

Which of these or others feel strongest for you?

____

____

____

____

Track Where This Fear Came From

Fear usually makes sense in context.

- ☐ Messages you received about epinephrine
- ☐ Past feelings of shame, dismissal, or confusion
- ☐ Misinformation that lingered
- ☐ Stories you heard from others
- ☐ A scary reaction in the past
- ☐ A bad experience with epinephrine

Write anything that comes to mind (even if it doesn't seem to make sense at first):

____

____

____

____

Separate Fear From Medical Guidance

Fear speaks loudly in emergencies, and makes it hard to follow sound medical guidance.

Fear says:

____

____

My allergist or medical team says:

____

____

What I know to be true about epinephrine:

____

____

Name a Compassionate Reframe

Complete this sentence compassionately:

When I hesitate, it does not mean I am failing. It means

____

____

Gradual Exposure to Reduce Needle Fear

 Needle fear is common among adults (Duncanson et al., 2021) and children (McMurtry et al., 2016) with chronic disease and can significantly interfere with treatment adherence and health outcomes. Exposure-based interventions are the most effective approach for managing high levels of needle fear across the lifespan. This approach helps the brain and body learn, over time, that something that feels scary can also be safe and manageable.

Gradual exposure works by breaking the experience into small, achievable steps. Each step is practiced repeatedly until it feels more comfortable before moving on to the next. The goal is not to eliminate fear right away, but to gradually build confidence and reduce how intense the fear feels over time.

This process can start with gentle exposure, such as looking at pictures or watching short videos of epinephrine being used, so the experience becomes more familiar. From there, you might move to practicing with a trainer device, holding the auto-injector, or walking through the steps of use without actually administering it. As comfort increases, the next steps could include watching a demonstration with a real device, observing someone else receive an injection, or practicing with an expired device on an orange. Over time, these small, repeated exposures can help the nervous system learn that this tool is safe, manageable, and something you can use effectively if needed.

Throughout this process, it is important to move at a pace that feels manageable. Repetition and nervous system regulation are key. Spending enough time at each step without pushing too far into the anxiety allows the nervous system to adjust and helps the experience feel less overwhelming. Actively supporting the nervous system with basic strategies like deep breathing, grounding exercises, and incorporating comfort and support can help. Over time, these small steps can lead to meaningful reductions in fear and increased confidence in handling medical procedures.

When to Seek Additional Support for Needle Phobia

Some fear is normal and may respond to the above ideas, but addressing needle phobia is beyond the scope of this workbook and may be addressed effectively by working with a professional. Professional support is recommended if you notice:

- Persistent panic attacks before appointments
- Avoidance of medically necessary care
- Refusal of injections or testing procedures despite strong desire for treatment
- Intense physical symptoms such as fainting
- Relationship conflict escalating around injection days
- Significant interference with work, school, sleep, eating, or any aspect of daily functioning

When needle fear begins to limit access to appropriate medical care, referral to a psychologist experienced in exposure-based treatment can be extremely effective. Needle phobia responds well to structured, gradual desensitization and nervous system regulation strategies.

Biologics represent a powerful new tool in food allergy care. Skin testing and blood draws may also be required to monitor treatment progress. Supporting the emotional experience alongside the medical treatment ensures that patients and families can actually sustain and benefit from what science now makes possible.

Working with Needle Fear

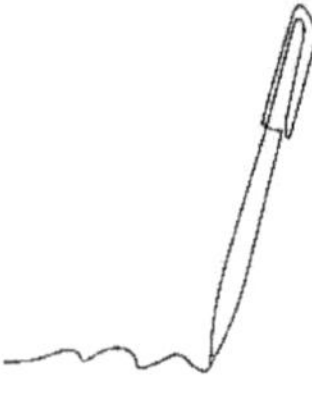

Use the following prompts to explore needle related anxiety.
Adult and teen patients or parents can complete this worksheet for themselves,
or use these questions to guide a conversation with their child.

Complete this page only if already exhibiting a strong fear of needles.

When I think about injections, the first thought that comes to mind is:

____

____

The worst thing I imagine happening is:

____

____

My body sensations before an injection usually include:

____

____

The level of fear I feel from 0 to 10 is (use a visual scale with faces or emojis with younger kids):

____

____

What evidence do I have that I can tolerate discomfort, even if I do not like it?

____

____

What coping strategy has helped me manage other fears successfully?

____

____

If this fear became smaller, what would that allow me to do or experience?

____

____

Helping Your Child Cope with Needle Fear

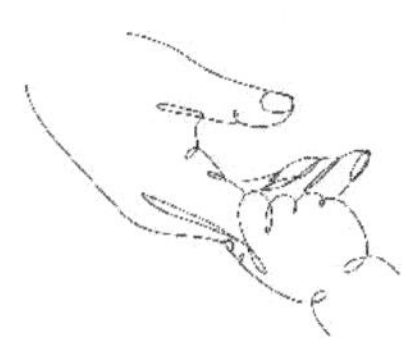

It is very common for children to feel nervous, scared, or even panicked about needles. For children managing food allergies or other medical needs, this fear can feel even bigger because injections may be part of staying safe.

The goal is not to eliminate fear completely, but to help your child move through the fear and build confidence with coping skills and support.

Notice Your Child's Starting Point

Take a moment to understand your child's current level of fear.

What situations cause distress?

☐ Talking about shots   ☐ Seeing pictures of needles   ☐ Being in medical settings

☐ Getting a shot themselves   ☐ Watching someone else get a shot   ☐ Other: ___________________

How does your child respond?

☐ Avoids or refuses   ☐ Cries or panics   ☐ Freezes or shuts down

☐ Asks repeated questions   ☐ Physical symptoms (e.g., stomachache, dizziness)

☐ Clings to you   ☐ Other: ____

Build a "Coping Toolbox"

Before discussing needles, help your child learn tools to calm their body.
Choose 2–3 strategies to learn and practice regularly when your child is calm:

☐ Counting or distraction games   ☐ Holding a comfort item and repeating affirmations

☐ Listening to music or a story   ☐ 4-7-8 breathing (in for 4, hold for 7, out for 8)

☐ Squeezing a stress ball   ☐ Guided imagery (e.g., imagining a safe place)

Use Role-Play to Build Confidence

For many children, practicing through play can reduce fear.

Use a toy medical kit and follow your child's lead as they explore the contents and different roles/scenarios. Invite your child to be the doctor and show what they think giving a shot looks and feels like, validate difficult emotions, model use of the coping strategies you've been practicing, and follow your child's lead while gently correcting misconceptions they may have that are evident in their play.

Don't forget to get silly to decrease the nervousness! You might pretend to be one of your child's favorite characters getting the shot, or express exaggerated silly misunderstandings about what getting a shot will involve and allow your child to correct and teach you. Remember that you are exploring emotions, not forcing them. Stay calm, validate feelings without getting into reassurance loops ("I promise it won't hurt"), and celebrate efforts and your time spent together.

Recognize When to Slow Down

If your child becomes overwhelmed, it may mean the step is too big.

If your child exhibits panic that does not settle, refusal to engage or shutdown, increased fear over time, or physical symptoms (dizziness, nausea):

- Return to an easier step

- Shorten practice time

- Increase support

When to Seek Additional Support

Consider professional support if:

- Fear is intense or worsening

- Medical care is being avoided

- Exposure practice is not helping

- Your child becomes highly distressed or panicked

A licensed mental health professional trained in trauma work and exposure therapy can provide structured, supportive guidance.

Reflection for Parents

What has your child done well?

____

____

What has been challenging?

____

____

What is one small next step?

____

____

Final Thought

Each small step helps you and your child learn:
"I can do hard things, even when I feel scared."

Additional Tips for Needle Fear

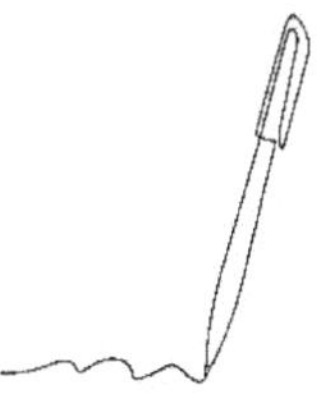

For some patients, the emotional challenge of injections is more daunting than the medication itself. The following strategies may help reduce pain and discomfort:

Supporting Physical Comfort
Reducing physical discomfort can help lower the intensity of the fear response:
☐ Apply a topical numbing cream as directed prior to injection
☐ Use a cold pack for a few minutes before and after to dull sensation
☐ Allow the medication to reach room temperature before administering (if permitted)
☐ Rotate injection sites to prevent irritation and sensitivity over time
☐ Use slow, steady pressure during the injection rather than rushing
☐ Consider using a vibration device near the injection site to help disrupt pain signals
☐ Recline/raise legs to support blood flow

Supporting the Nervous System
Help the nervous system learn over time that the experience is safe and manageable:
☐ Practice paced breathing before and during the injection (slow inhale, longer exhale)
☐ Use guided imagery, such as imagining a calming or familiar place
☐ Listen to music, a favorite show, or a story during the process
☐ Keep your body as relaxed as possible, especially the injection site
☐ Use grounding techniques, such as noticing what you can see, hear, or feel around you

Building Predictability and Routine
Consistency can significantly reduce anticipatory anxiety:
☐ Pair injections with a predictable routine (same time, same setting when possible)
☐ Talk through the steps ahead of time so there are no surprises
☐ Keep supplies organized and easily accessible
☐ Use the same sequence each time to create a sense of familiarity

Increasing Control and Participation
Participation helps shift the experience from something happening *to* them into something they are actively navigating.
☐ Offer choices where possible, even small ones
☐ Allow distraction if helpful (off-topic discussion or other activity like music or a video)
☐ Practice with a trainer device or role-play the steps ahead of time
☐ Encourage communication about preferences for what helps or doesn't
☐ Involve children in age-appropriate ways (choose the location, hold supplies, count down)

Needle fear does not disappear overnight. With repetition, support, and small, intentional steps, it often becomes more manageable. The goal is not to eliminate discomfort completely, but to help the body and mind learn that this is something you can move through with increasing confidence.

Getting Comfortable with Epinephrine

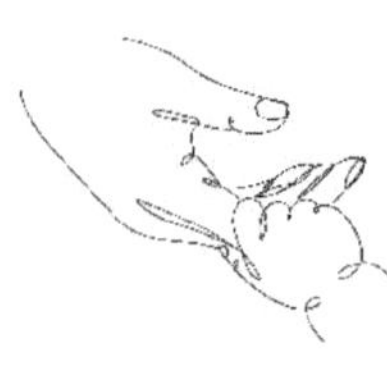

For many children, epinephrine feels big, scary, and mysterious. They hear adults talk about emergencies, reactions, and "just in case," but often without everyday, calm conversation to make it feel familiar. When something is only discussed during stressful moments, children's nervous systems often learn that the topic itself is dangerous, shameful, scary, or taboo.

One of the best ways to reduce fear is through ordinary, low-pressure exposure. When we incorporate epinephrine into everyday conversation and play, we help children build familiarity instead of fear. The goal is not to make epinephrine feel casual or unimportant, but to make it feel understandable, manageable, and less overwhelming.

Children learn best through repetition, play, and safe connection. Make epinephrine part of normal life instead of something that only appears during fear.

Simple, Confident Language

Use everyday moments to talk calmly about epinephrine in small, manageable pieces. Avoid turning the conversation into something overly dramatic. Calm confidence helps children borrow your sense of safety.

This is your epinephrine. It is medicine that helps your body if you have a serious allergic reaction.

Epinephrine helps keep you safe.

Let Them See It and Hold It

Show your child the real epinephrine device, and let them hold and play with a trainer device. Be sure to explain that the trainer has no medicine and is made just for practice and play. If you don't have a trainer, ask your allergist or request one through the device manufacturer's website.

Let them look at it, ask questions, and watch how it is administered. If you aren't sure, watch a video online before discussing with your child. Emphasize that the medicine would help them feel better if they ever needed it, other safety steps that would be taken to care for them, and point out which helpers and caregivers would help them so they would feel better quickly.

Practice Through Play

Children often process fear through play long before they can talk about it directly. Keep the epinephrine trainers in a toy medical kit and get this and toy food out for occasional play. If your child isn't interested, prompt them with ideas like the child being a doctor or nurse, teaching a stuffed animal or doll to use epinephrine, playing restaurant, packing a bag for school or a trip, etc.

Follow your child's lead. Play often tells you what they are thinking.

Getting Comfortable with Dosing Tools

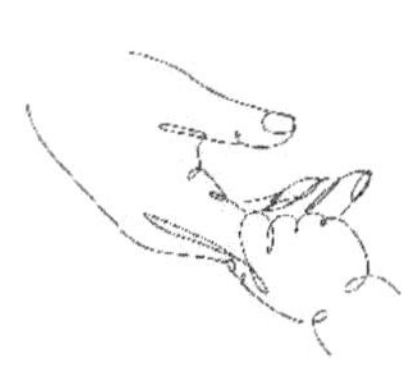 New medical equipment can feel unfamiliar or even scary, even when they are not painful. This activity helps your child become comfortable through play, practice, and predictability. Ask your doctor about any equipment that will be used (syringes, blood pressure cuff, stethoscope, pulse oximeter, spirometer, etc.) and incorporate it into play.

We'll use the example of an oral syringe, since children often mistake these for needles, but you can use play to decrease anxiety around any aspect of care.

Introduce the Tool

Show your child the oral syringe. Emphasize that there is no needle.

You might say: "This is a tool that helps us measure your dose. It's not a shot. It doesn't poke."

Let them hold it, explore it, and ask questions.

Practice with Water

Fill the syringe with a few drops of colored water or a drink your child enjoys to motivate them. Practice dosing based on your treatment plan.

For OIT or SLIT (swallowing):
Gently place the syringe in the mouth. Slowly push the liquid in. Practice holding under tongue/swallowing. Do this yourself first, then invite your child to try it.

For SLIT (under the tongue):
Place the liquid under the tongue. Hold for the recommended time. Spit it out. Be silly!
Invite your child to copy you.

Get Playful

To reduce fear and build familiarity, let your child give you, a pet, or a stuffed animal a "dose."

Get silly: squirt water, make a mess, laugh, experiment. Shift the unknown to something fun.

Recreate the Appointment

If possible, ask your provider ahead of time what the first visit will be like.

Then set up a "pretend appointment" at home. Practice sitting, waiting, dosing.

Include any steps your child will experience, and photos of the office areas if possible.

Ask Open-Ended Questions

Ask your child neutral things like: What did you think? How was it?

Validate any feelings that come up, and write down any questions your child might have.

Create a Plan

Give your child age-appropriate choices. Options might include:

Holding a toy, sitting close to you, having a distraction, or even doing their own dose if old enough

Write or draw the plan here:

Children often fear what they don't understand or haven't experienced, and they learn best through silliness and play. When they can see, touch, practice, and play with something new, it becomes far less scary.

Immunotherapy Progress Map

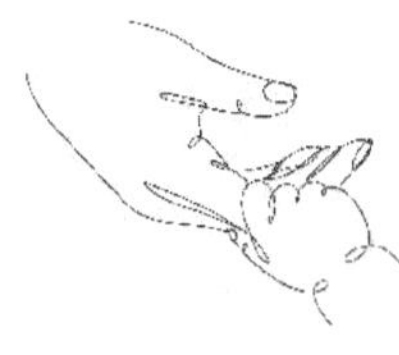 This page will help you plan ways to support your child in seeing the journey, making it fun, and staying motivated. Use this page to track progress with your child, or plan a different way to help them grasp the bigger picture, get invested and excited, and stay motivated long term. It is helpful to create a visual way to mark progress, celebrate milestones, and create meaning along the way.

Getting Started

The pages that follow are meant to be copied and cut out to build a path or map. As you progress, you'll build the road and complete the blank signs to mark progress, highlights, and milestones. Get creative and add additional drawings or stickers to represent any moment you may want to acknowledge, big or small.

These might include:

- Starting treatment

- Completing an up-dose

- Trying a new form of a food

- Getting through a hard day

- Returning to dosing after a break or reaction

- Reaching maintenance

- Or any personal milestone that matters to you or your child

There is no "right" way to use the map, only what feels meaningful for your journey.

Make It Your Own

Your child can color the map and add "stickers" from the included page to mark milestones and create a visual story of their adventure. Encourage your child to personalize it in any way that feels fun and engaging by using your own stickers, adding drawings or photos, and adding reflections.

Making this interactive and creative can help build a sense of pride, ownership, and motivation.

Use as Many Pages as You Need

This will probably not be a one-page journey.

You are encouraged to copy this page as many times as needed and expand your map as you go. Some patients may not need much space, and others may need more.

Find a place to assemble and display the map as it winds and grows as a visual reminder. This might be on a large piece of posterboard, on the back of a door, on your refrigerator, or on a tack board.

Create Your Own System

If this format doesn't quite fit your child's personality or interests, have fun creating your own version of a progress tracker.

Some ideas:

- A sticker chart with a favorite theme (animals, sports, space, favorite characters)

- A "leveling up" system (like a video game)

- A journal or logbook

- A visual timeline on a wall or poster

The goal is to make progress *visible* and *celebrated* in a way that feels exciting and meaningful for your child.

A Gentle Reminder

Progress in immunotherapy is not always linear.

Some days will feel like big steps forward. Others may feel slower, harder, or uncertain. Every step counts, and every effort matters.

It is important to create a fun way to remind yourself and your child how far you've come.

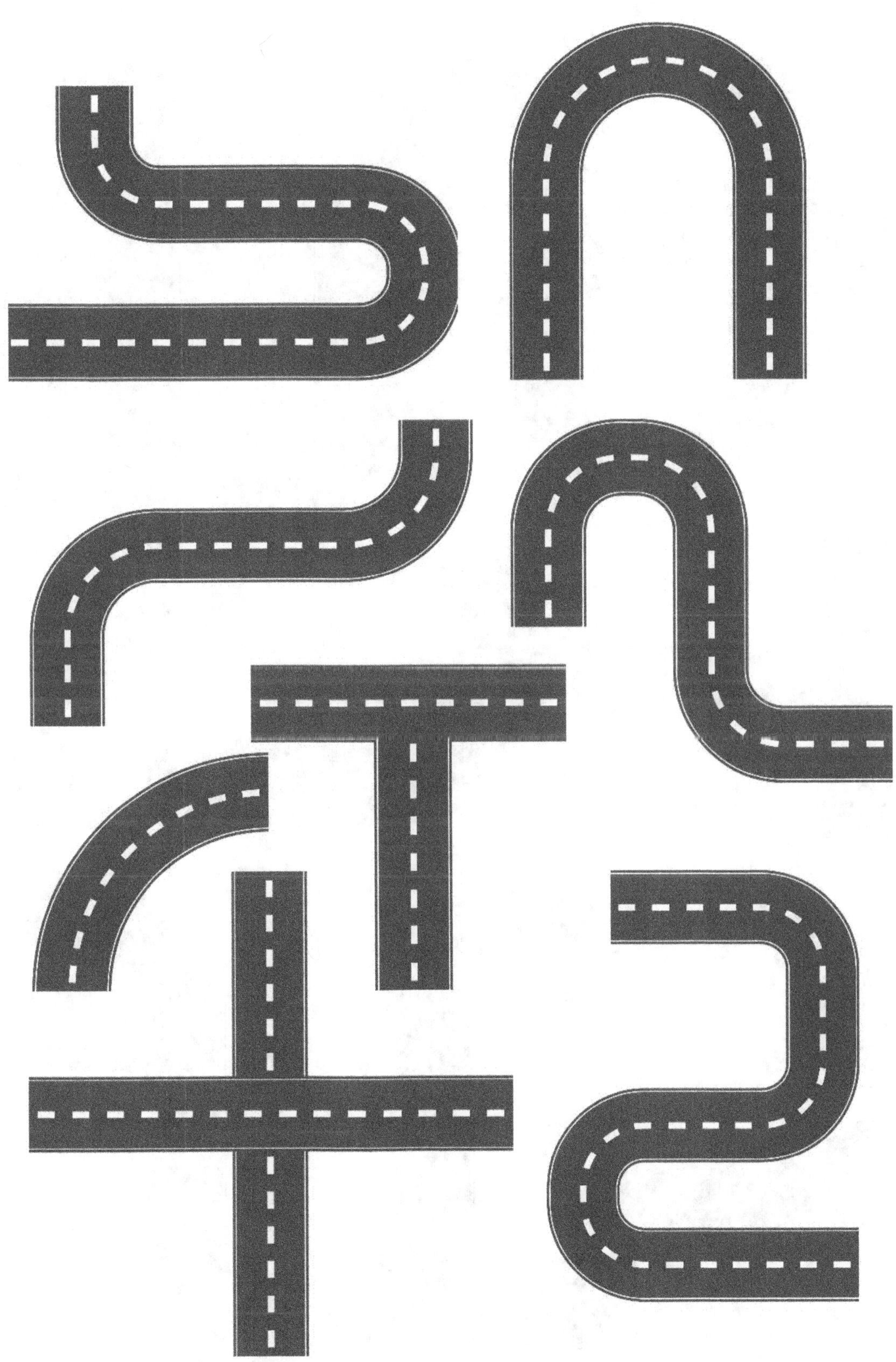

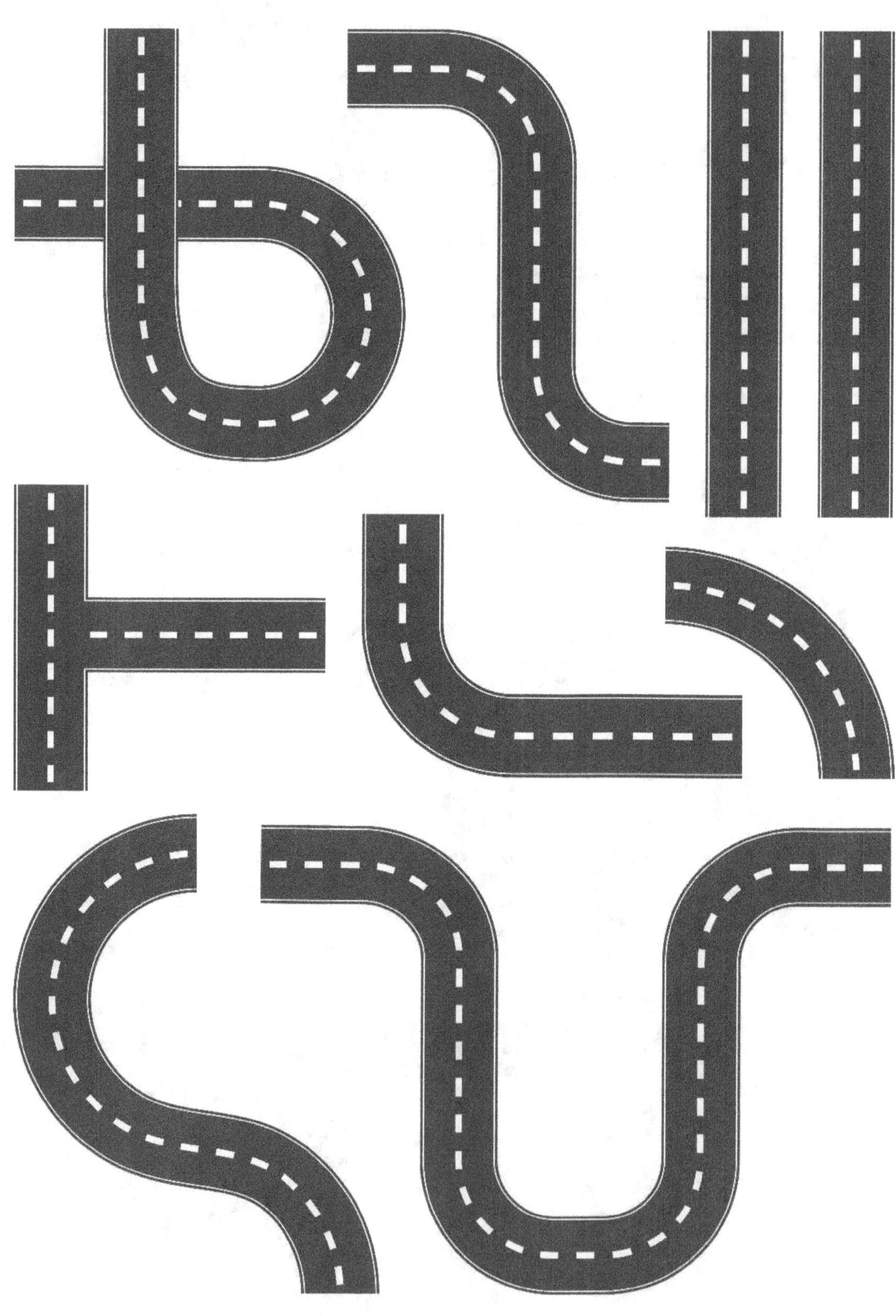

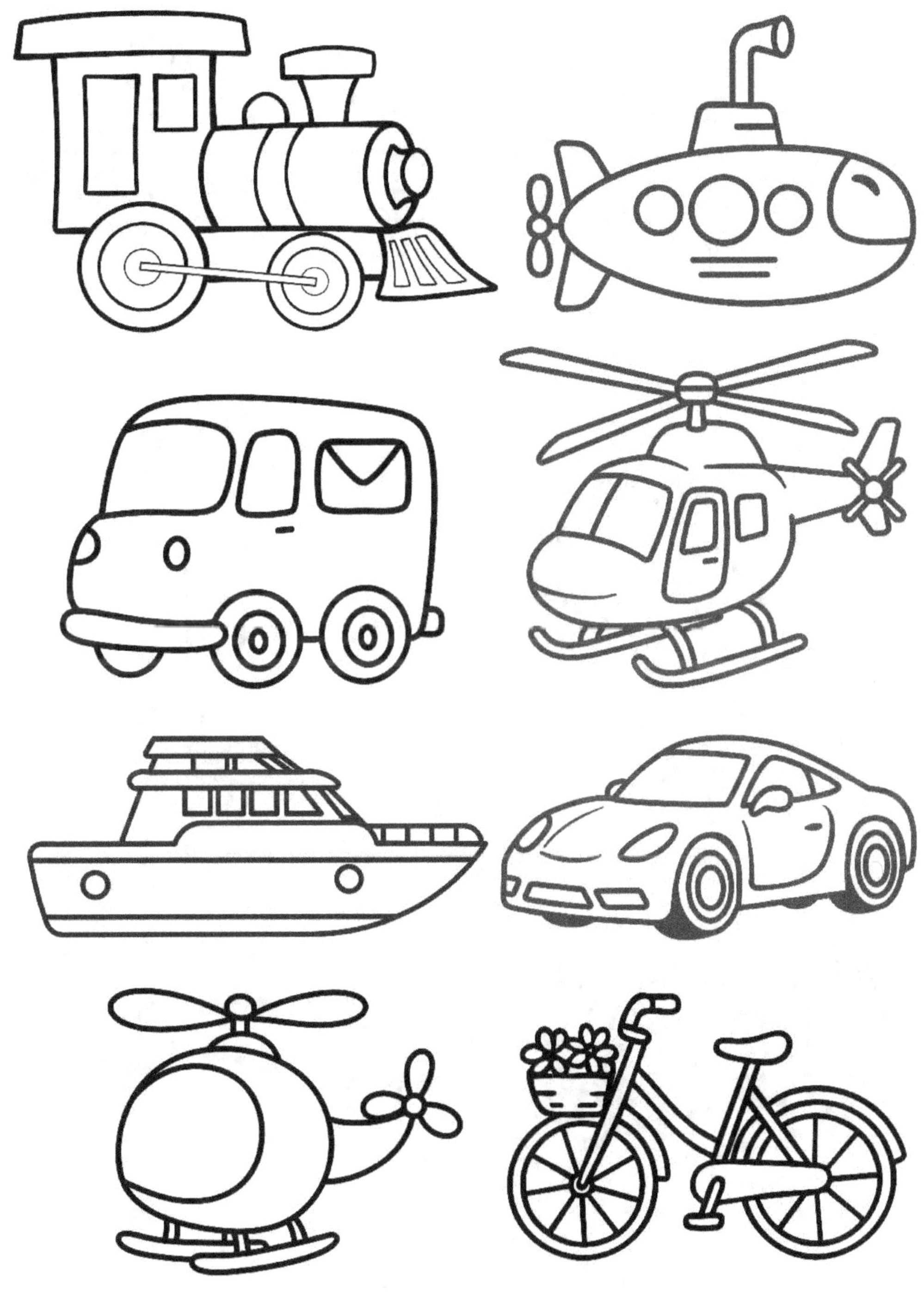

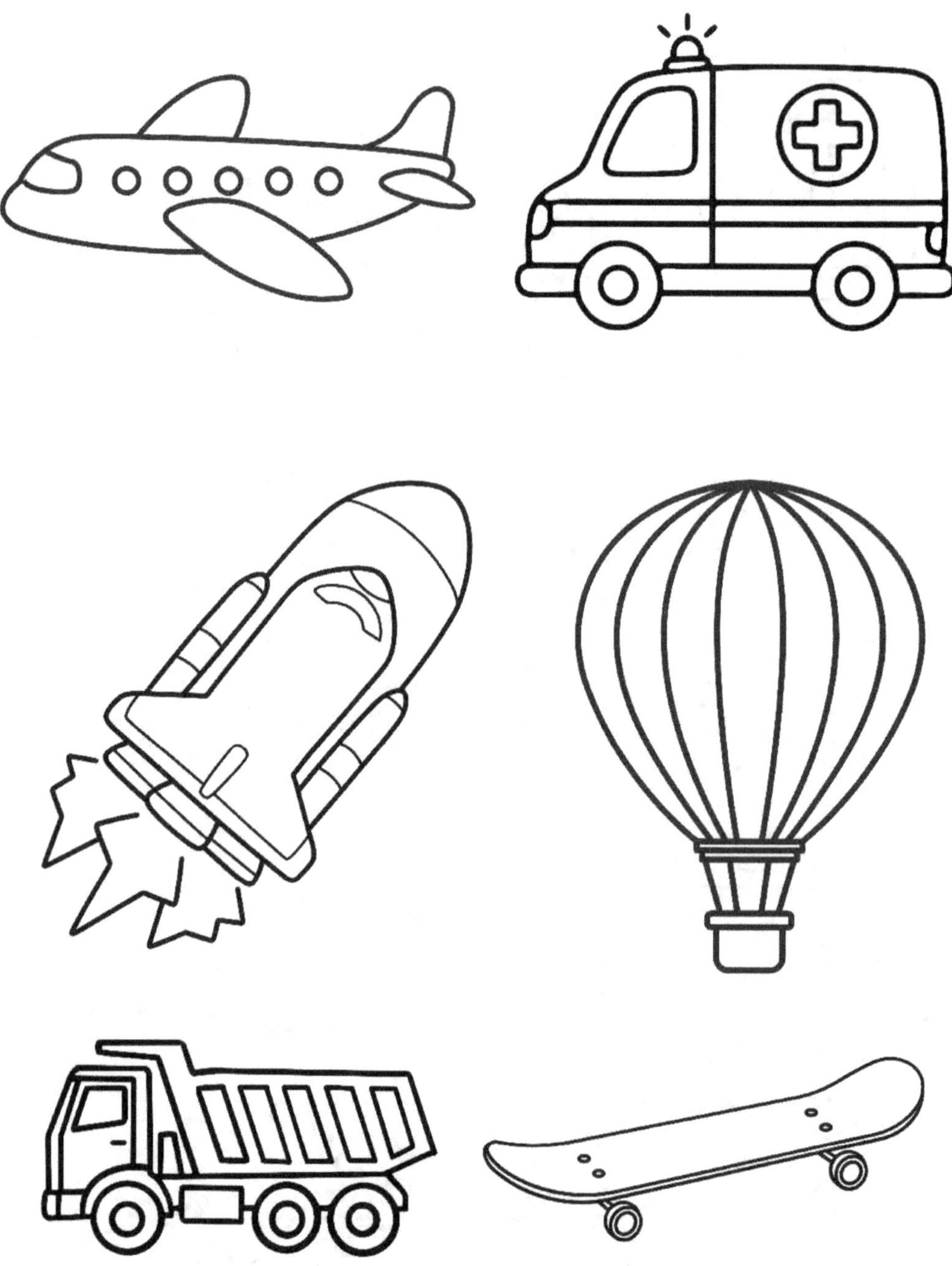

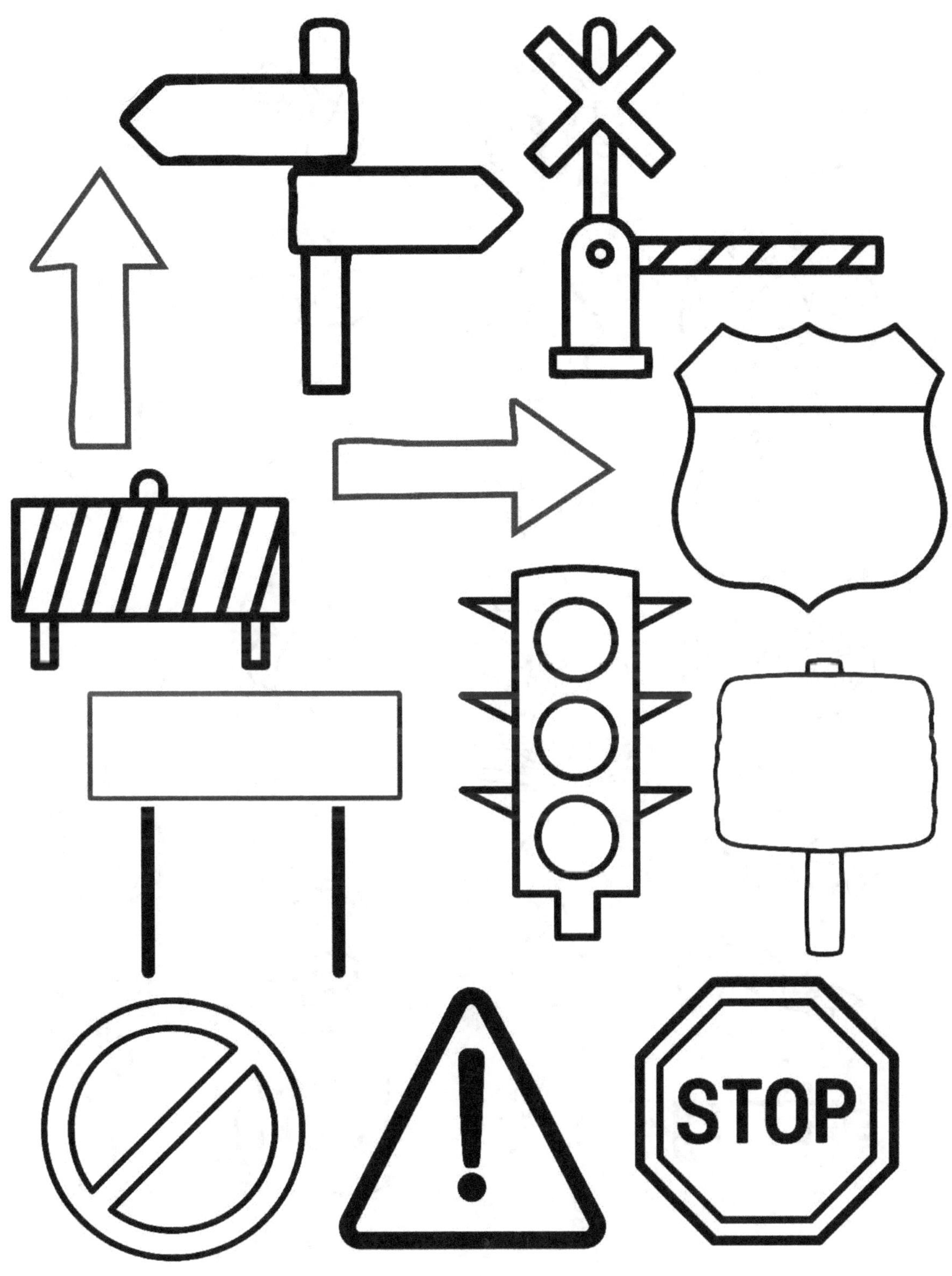

Part V:
Hitting the Road

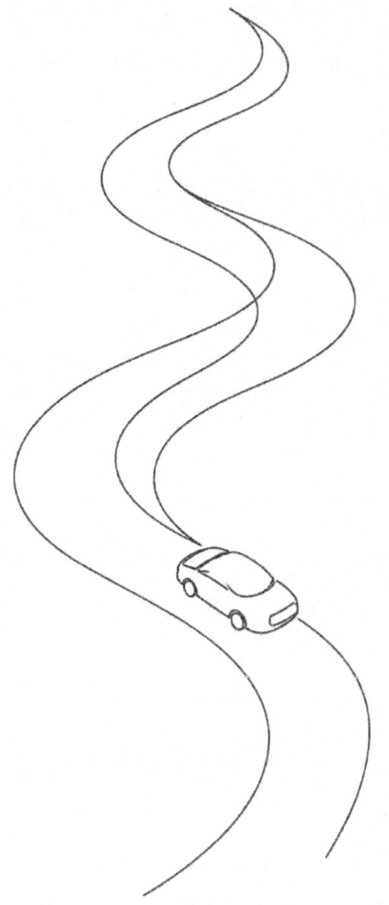

The most difficult thing is the decision to act,

the rest is merely tenacity.

— Amelia Earhart

Chapter 8:
Starting Out

In the days leading up to our OIT start date, I was full of nervous energy. I am someone who copes by staying busy, and preparing for the appointment gave me a long list of tasks that helped channel that energy. I packed for the appointment itself and prepared our two other children as well. The night before, we drove to my parents' house in Pennsylvania, stayed overnight, and left the younger kids there during the day so my son and I could go to the doctor together.

When I felt anxious, I found myself replaying my earlier conversations with the physician in my mind. I remembered his calm, confident voice and the moment I had decided that I would have to trust him. Of course, I was still afraid of the worst case scenario: a severe reaction. The fact that the clinic was attached to a hospital was reassuring, at least on a practical level. What helped more emotionally was shifting our focus to the best case scenario. My son and I revisited the goals we had set for treatment, including his very specific hope of being able to eat a donut at a certain popular Buffalo spot without worrying about cross contact.

Once we arrived, we settled into a corner of the waiting room, knowing we would be there for quite a while. In another corner, another mother and son were doing the same. We soon realized it was their first day of OIT as well. We became fast friends, encouraging the kids to share the activities they had brought and quietly talking with each other when the boys were distracted. That sense of connection and mutual understanding was one of the most meaningful parts of the day. I remember her explaining that her son was an athlete who had chosen to pause competing for a year so he could pursue treatment, with the hope of having more freedom in his sport long term.

My son's initial dosing went well. He loved the purple Kool Aid and was thrilled by the extra video game time and snacks while we waited. The staff were warm, cheerful, organized, reassuring, and confident. I watched him closely, trying to look casually interested in his game while actually monitoring his breathing, his posture, his eyes, and his ears, scanning for any sign of a reaction. Every small movement caught my attention as I tried to determine whether it was normal restlessness or the beginning of symptoms.

The doses were given in small increments. When my son's ear became slightly red and puffy, something that had historically been associated with his reactions, we stopped for the day. It was that simple! When I pointed it out, I realized I had been bracing myself for pushback or dismissal. Instead, the team simply noted it and adjusted accordingly. He did not need any medications. The dose prior to the one that made his ear red became the starting dose we left the office with that day.

We drove back to my parents' house, relieved by how uneventful the day had been. That night, after we all went to sleep, my son woke up coughing. Earlier in our journey, I would not have known that a cough alone could signal a reaction, but by then I was highly sensitized to it. I called the clinic's emergency number, and our doctor answered. He advised us to give oral antihistamines, monitor closely, and use epinephrine if any additional symptoms appeared or if the cough did not resolve. He stayed in contact with us by text until everything settled, which it did.

The next day, we spoke again and discussed the fact that my parents have a cat, to which my son is allergic. He had already started SLIT for his environmental allergies for this reason, but those take time to work. The doctor eased my mind by reminding me that the at-home dose was lower than the dose that had caused the ear swelling at the office, and encouraged us to dose that day.

Although our original plan had been to rely on my parents' support so my husband could join us for the long trips and updose appointments, we adjusted. If I learned anything through this process, it is the importance of flexibility. Make a plan, and be prepared to change the plan. I had to change a major part of our plan on Day 1, but we made it work.

Beginning Treatment: What This Phase Really Is

You may have spent weeks, months, or even years gathering information, weighing options, and imagining what this might be like. This moment often surprises people, not because they are unprepared, but because of how intense it can feel. Even when the decision is thoughtful, the treatment is appropriate, and hope is present, the experience of starting can feel bigger than expected. If that is true for you, you are not alone, and you are not doing anything wrong.

At the beginning of treatment, many people expect to feel reassured by the structure, the supervision, and the medical guidance. What might also show up is activation. You might notice a racing mind, a tight chest, a heightened awareness of every sensation, or a sudden urge to double-check, research more, or change your mind. This is not a sign that something is wrong. It is a sign that your nervous system is doing exactly what it was designed to do.

From a nervous system perspective, food allergies are not abstract. They are learned experiences of threat. Over time, the brain becomes highly efficient at detecting and responding to anything that might resemble risk. Even though you are beginning treatment in a controlled, medically supervised environment, your brain may interpret this as doing something that has not been safe before. That response is protective, not pathological.

Symptoms as Positive Signals

One of the most challenging aspects of starting immunotherapy is observing closely for signs of a reaction, the very thing most of us fear the most. Learning how to interpret symptoms is a key skill that we must develop. Mild symptoms such as itching, tingling, irritated skin, or slight gastrointestinal discomfort can occur. For individuals and families who have been trained to respond quickly to any sign of a reaction, these sensations can feel alarming. However, emerging research has helped reframe this experience in a more helpful and more calming way. The research team at Stanford University has demonstrated that when patients are taught how to view these mild, non-emergency symptoms as "positive signals," their emotional state and treatment outcomes improve (Howe et al., 2019). Suggesting that mild, transient symptoms can sometimes reflect the immune system engaging with treatment and adapting appears to empower and reassure patients and families.

Of course, this does not mean that symptoms should be ignored, nor does it replace medical guidance or emergency protocols. Instead, it offers an important shift in perspective: not every sensation means something is wrong. Some sensations mean something is happening. Learning to distinguish between signals of adaptation and signals of true risk is a process that takes time, support, and repeated experience.

Sensation Reframing

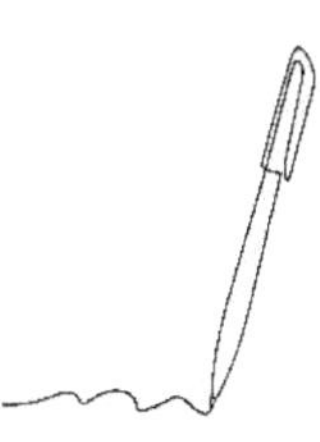

During immunotherapy, many people notice physical sensations that can easily be interpreted as warning signs or threats. This page helps you gently examine how you describe those sensations and practice reframing them in ways that are accurate, regulated, and supportive. This is not about ignoring symptoms or pushing through discomfort. The goal is to develop a shared, medically informed language that reduces unnecessary fear and supports nervous system regulation.

Name What You Notice

List sensations you've noticed during or after dosing. These may be familiar patterns or one-off experiences. Examples might include things like: warmth in ears, itchy tongue, stomach sensations

____

____

Language Audit

Notice the words you use internally or aloud when these sensations appear. Ask yourself: What words do I use _in my head?_ What words do I say out loud to my child, partner, or provider? Do these words escalate fear, or do they create space for observation?

____

____

Meaning-Making (With Your Care Team)

For each sensation, note what your medical team has advised _in your specific case._ Reframing is collaborative, should incorporate your provider's feedback, and should never dismiss safety.

____

____

Emotional Impact Check

Notice how language influences your emotional response. How does your body feel when you use threat-based language compared to when you use neutral language?

____

____

Choose a Practice Phrase

Select one or two phrases you want to intentionally practice using going forward. (Examples: "This sensation has shown up before and passed, " "Noticing doesn't automatically mean danger. "

____

____

Notice and Color

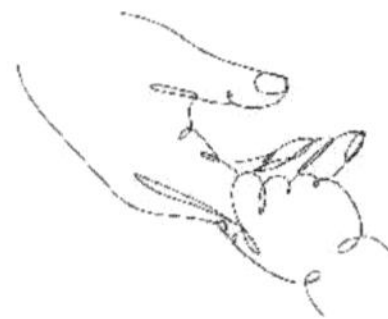 Sometimes bodies feel things during immunotherapy. This activity helps children show what they notice without labeling it as "good" or "bad." Noticing is something bodies do. It does not always mean danger.

This activity is recommended for children who are expressing worry or concern about any symptoms they are noticing during immunotherapy. If your child is not reporting apprehension, it is likely best not to draw attention to any signals in the body.

Materials

- Choose a body outline from the following pages
- Crayons, colored pencils, or markers
- Optional: stickers, stamps, or dot markers

Introduce the Idea

Use calm, neutral language.

"Sometimes your body notices your dose. Noticing means your body is paying attention and your immune system is learning to respond in a new way. We're going to color what your body notices."

Choose Colors for Sensations

Invite the child to decide what different colors mean *to them*. If helpful, they may use lighter/darker shades or lighter/darker coloring strokes to show smaller and bigger sensations.

Color the Body

Prompt gently, and let your child lead without correcting them.

- "Can you color where your body noticed something today?"
- "Did any spots feel warm, tingly, itchy, or funny?"
- "Are there places with no color at all?"

Intensity Without Fear

If a child colors something dark or large, respond with curiosity, not alarm. This reinforces that sensations change, bodies regulate, and adults are calm and available.

"That looks like a strong noticing. Strong doesn't always mean dangerous. What happened next?"

Normalize & Name

Choose words that fit your child's age and temperament.

- "Your body noticed—and it stayed safe."
- "Noticing is how your body learns."
- "This is information, not an emergency."
- "Your body is practicing."

Optional:

Let the child add:

- A checkmark for sensations that went away
- A star for "things my body handled"
- A speech bubble with what their body might say
  (e.g., *"I'm learning"* or *"I noticed and then relaxed"*)

Notes about your child's comments or observations:

____

____

____

____

____

Closing

Thank you for showing me what your body noticed. We'll keep noticing together and take care of you as a team.

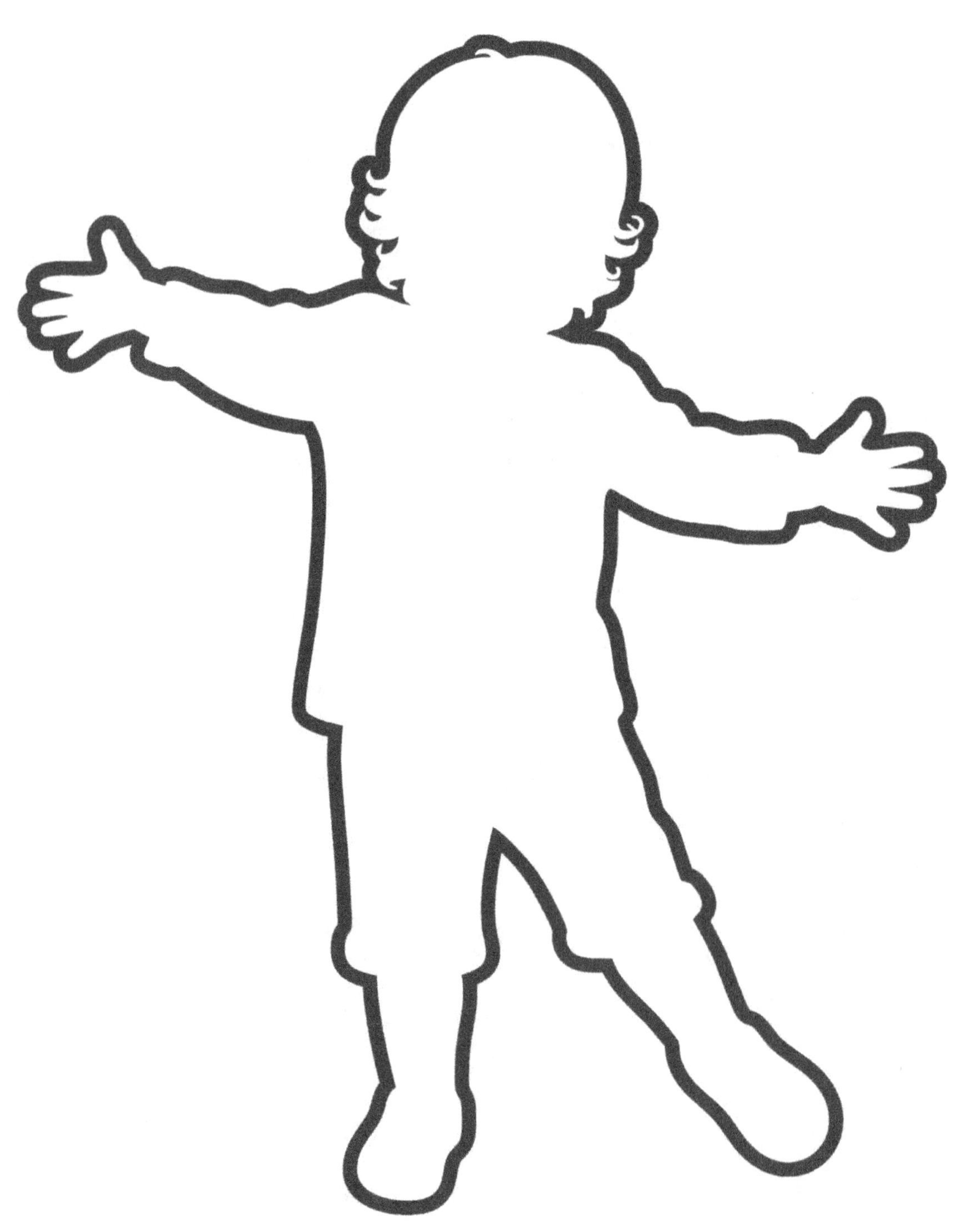

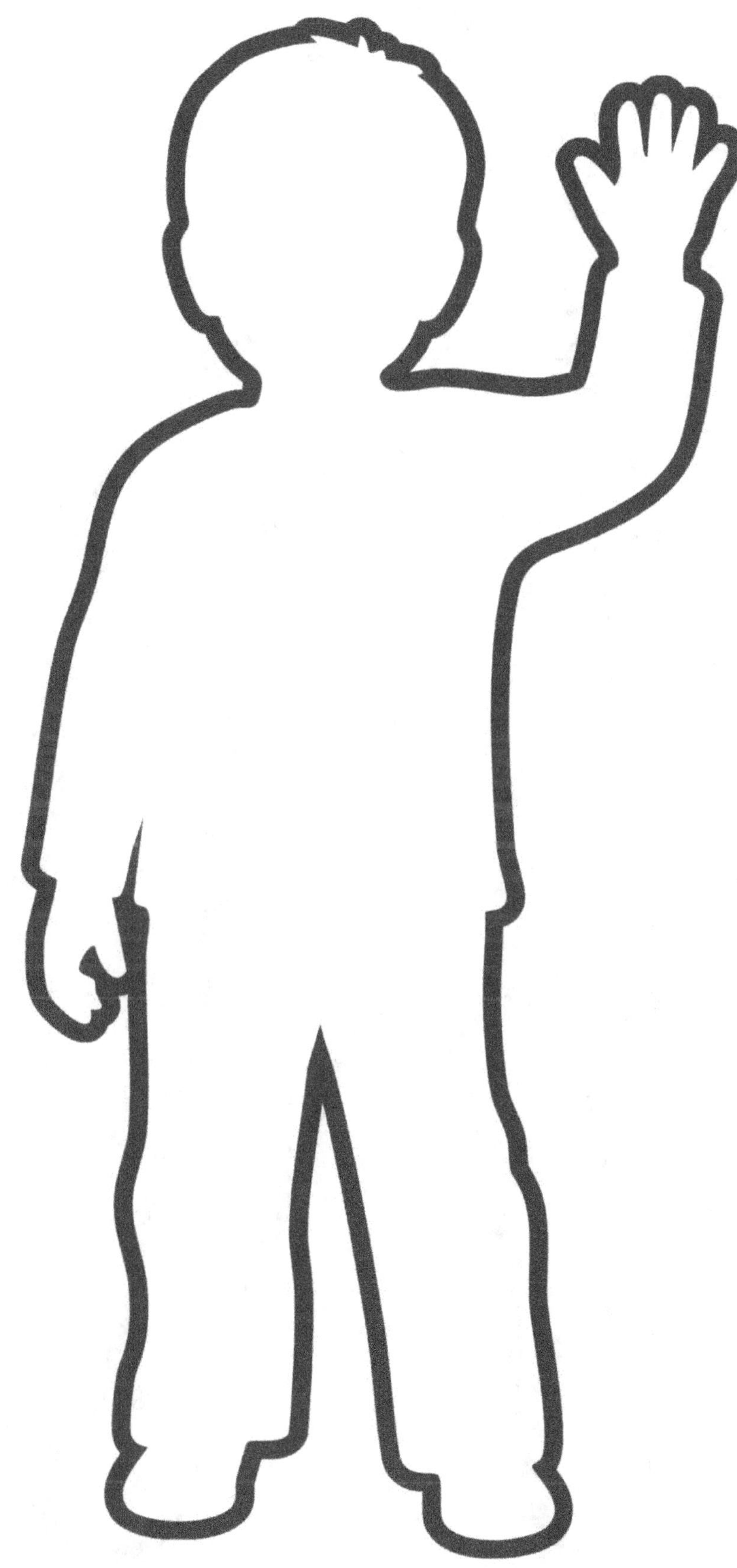

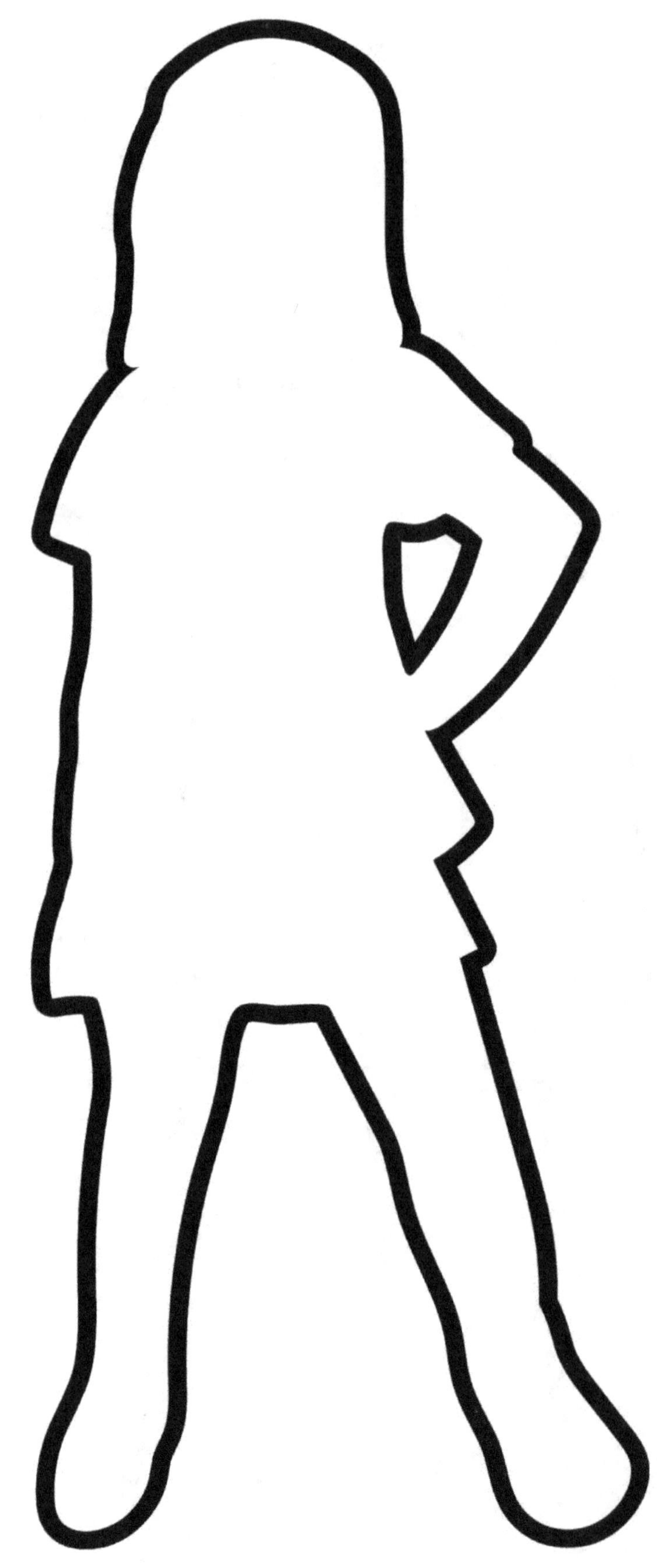

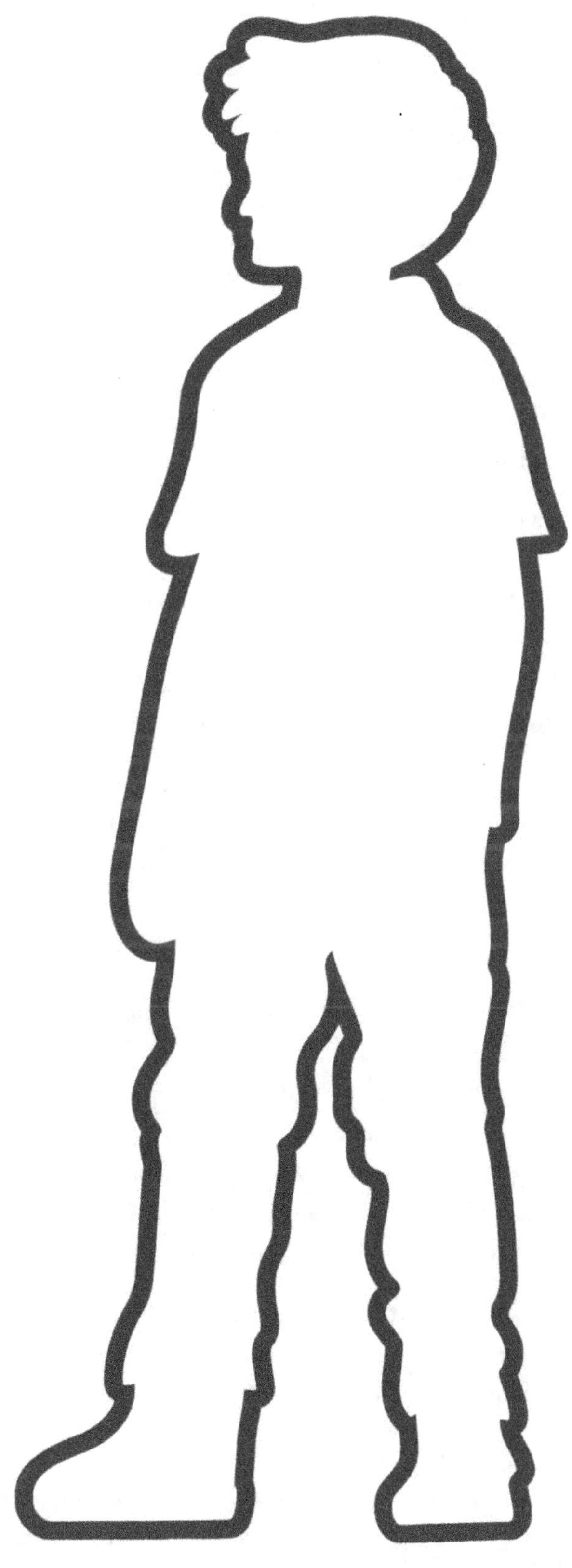

Chapter 9:
Logging the Miles

Normalizing the Emotional Experience

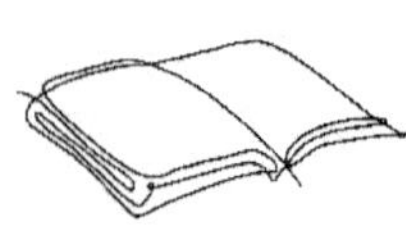 It is common to assume that feeling anxious means you are not ready. In reality, fear and hope often exist side by side. You may feel hopeful about increased safety and freedom while also feeling afraid of what it will take to get there. You may feel confident in your decision and still question it in quieter moments.

These are not contradictions; they are part of the same process. When something matters and carries uncertainty, the mind naturally moves between approaching and pulling away. That tension does not mean you should stop. It means this is meaningful and important to you.

Many find that starting treatment is the hardest part because of the anticipation. Before the first dose, everything is unknown, and the mind fills in the gaps with worst-case scenarios. After the first few doses, patterns begin to emerge. Expectations become grounded in lived experience, and confidence starts to build. Over time, what once felt overwhelming often becomes routine. This reflects what we know about learning and exposure: repeated, safe experiences gradually reshape the brain's threat response (Craske et al., 2014). At the beginning, before those experiences accumulate, your brain fills the space with caution.

It is important to understand that there is no version of this process in which you are supposed to feel calm from the start. You are not behind if you feel anxious, if you second-guess, if you need reassurance, or if you move more slowly than you expected. You are responding as a human being navigating something meaningful and uncertain.

Common Emotional Patterns

While each experience is unique, there are common emotional patterns that often emerge at the beginning of treatment. Anticipatory anxiety may show up before appointments or doses, bringing thoughts about what might happen or how things could go. Catastrophic thinking can follow, with the mind jumping to worst-case scenarios as a way of trying to prepare. Hypervigilance may lead you to closely monitor your body or your child's body, noticing every sensation and change. This level of awareness can feel exhausting, but it shows up because it has helped keep you safe in the past. Over time, as new and safe experiences accumulate, this vigilance can begin to soften.

You may also notice a tension between control and uncertainty. Before treatment, safety may have come from strict avoidance, clear rules, and predictable routines. Beginning treatment can feel like stepping into something less familiar, even though it is medically structured. It can feel like changing something that has kept you safe.

Children often look to their caregivers to interpret what is happening. If a parent feels anxious, even subtly, a child may sense that something is not safe. This does not mean you need to eliminate your own anxiety. Instead, it highlights the importance of co-regulation. Staying present and steady together, naming your emotions, and modeling positive coping skills when experiences feel challenging teaches our children resilience.

Helpful Strategies

Certain thoughts tend to arise frequently during this phase. You might find yourself asking, "What if something goes wrong?" While this question reflects a natural concern, it can be helpful to gently remind yourself that you are not unprepared. You are entering a process with medical guidance, clear protocols, and tools to respond if needed. This is not unmanaged risk; it is supported exposure.

You might also wonder, "What if I made the wrong decision?" In those moments, it can help to return to the reality that you made the best decision you could with the information, values, and support you had at the time. If you completed worksheets in the decision-making chapter, it may be helpful to revisit those and your frame of thinking at that time. Decisions are not judged by outcomes alone, and you can continue to reassess as you move forward. Another common thought is, "We were safe before. Why risk it?" While avoidance can provide a form of safety, it likely came with limitations for you if you chose to pursue immunotherapy. In other words, if you chose immunotherapy, there was a reason. In this moment, treatment might feel like you are abandoning safety, but it is really about expanding safety.

Predictable routines can reduce uncertainty by creating consistency around dosing and expectations. A clear understanding of what to expect, including which symptoms are typical and which require action, can help reduce fear. Limiting over-researching can prevent the mind from becoming overwhelmed, as more information does not always lead to greater reassurance. Building trust with providers by asking questions and clarifying plans can also provide a sense of stability. Trust is not immediate. It develops over time through experience.

The next pages will help you slow down, reflect, and step into this starting point with greater clarity, so that wherever this path leads, you are not just moving forward, but moving forward with awareness.

Marking the Beginning

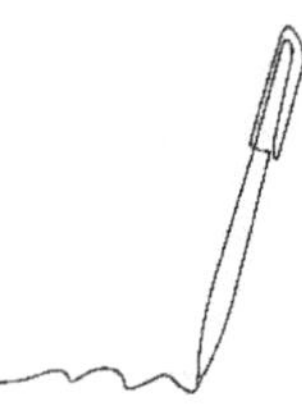

Starting treatment is a meaningful transition no matter how it went. This page is not about evaluating the day as "good" or "bad," but about noticing, honoring, and marking the moment you began and however you feel about it.

Take a Moment to Pause

You've taken a step that may have felt big, uncertain, hopeful, overwhelming, or all of these at once. Before jumping back into your busy routine, give yourself a moment to acknowledge: You started.

Reflect on Your Experience

There is no right or wrong way for this day to have gone. Use the space below to reflect honestly and without judgment.

What stands out most from today?

____

____

What surprised you (in any direction)?

____

____

What felt easier than you expected?

____

____

What felt harder than you expected?

____

____

Other reflections:

____

____

____

____

____

Name What You Carried Into Today

My thoughts going into this were:

____

____

One feeling I noticed was:

____

____

Name What You're Carrying Forward

One thing I learned from today:

____

____

One thing I want to remember for next time:

____

____

Mark the Moment

Choose one small, intentional way to acknowledge this transition. You might:

☐ Share a quiet moment with someone together after the appointment

☐ Celebrate with a favorite meal, dessert, or drink

☐ Take a photo

☐ Talk to someone you trust about the experience

☐ Go somewhere familiar or comforting

☐ Say something simple out loud like, "I/we did it"

Write what you chose (or plan to choose):

____

____

____

____

____

The Journey Begins

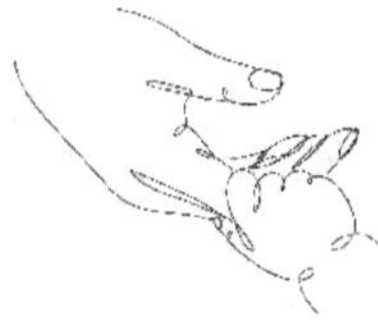 Children process experiences through play, not just conversation. This activity allows them to revisit the appointment in a way that feels safe, familiar, and within their control. You don't need to "teach" anything in this moment. Just be present.

Gather simple items and let your child choose what to use:

A toy doctor kit or household substitutes

A small cup, spoon, or syringe (real or pretend)

Stuffed animals or dolls

Follow Your Child's Lead

Invite your child to "play the appointment," but do not direct or correct.

You might say: *Do you want to show me/Dad/your brother what it was like today?*

Your child may replay what happened, change parts of the story, focus on specific moments.

Join Gently

If your child invites you in, take on any role that they want you to.

Many children want to be the doctor and give you a "dose" for a sense of control and mastery.

Others will simply release silly energy that is unrelated to the day.

Reflect Without Leading

Give simple reflections using the same words your child chooses.

Speak in short phrases that help them feel seen:

That part felt big. You remembered that. You helped your bear do it.

Avoid correcting or adding new information unless your child asks or leads the way.

Optional Gentle Prompts

If your child seems talkative, you might ask open-ended questions like:

What was your favorite part? What felt a little tricky? What helped you?

Closing the Activity

You might end by thanking them for showing you, noticing something they did well, or following their lead to a different activity.

Write down anything that stood out or that you'd like to remember:

____

____

____

Chapter 10:
Traveling Together

Getting Caregivers on Board for Treatment

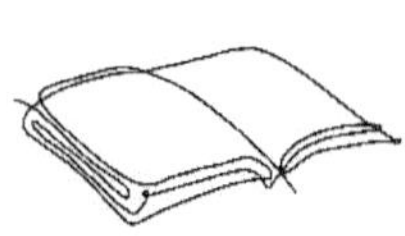 One of the more complex parts of starting treatment is how to communicate about it with caregivers outside the home. Food allergy care is often understood in simple terms: avoid the allergen and be prepared to respond to a reaction. Immunotherapy adds nuance. A child who is actively ingesting their allergen as part of treatment is still allergic and may require even more structured support around dosing times, rest periods, or activity restrictions.

This can be confusing for others, especially if they are used to thinking about food allergies in more black-and-white terms. One common challenge is misunderstanding. For example, if a child shares that they are "eating their allergen now," it may be interpreted as the allergy being resolved, which can lead to relaxed precautions.

Because of this, families often need to carefully consider how much to share and with whom. Some choose to keep details minimal, especially if treatment happens entirely at home and does not affect time in another caregiver's setting. Others may need to communicate more directly if care routines, supervision, or activity need to be adjusted. This may be necessary if:

- dosing occurs before school and requires a rest period that overlaps with the school day

- activity restrictions (such as delaying gym or recess) are needed

- symptoms may need to be monitored in the school setting

There is no single correct approach. The goal is to find a balance between clarity, safety, and practicality for your specific situation. When communication is needed, clarity and simplicity are most helpful. Focus on what the caregiver needs to know to keep your child safe:

- Your child is still allergic

- All usual safety precautions remain in place

- Treatment involves controlled exposure under medical guidance

- Any specific instructions (e.g., timing, supervision, activity limits)

Equally important is helping your child understand these same rules. Immunotherapy can be confusing for kids because they may eat their allergen(s) at home but still need to follow strict safety precautions elsewhere. Preparing your child for how to talk about their treatment can reduce confusion for them and others. Children are often proud of their progress and may share it in simple terms that others misunderstand. Giving them language that is both accurate and age-appropriate helps others understand while maintaining appropriate safety.

Caregiver Communication Planning Sheet

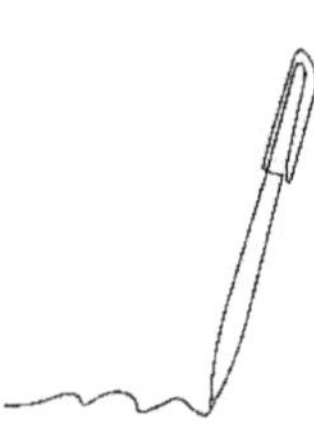

Communicating about your child's treatment with caregivers outside the home can feel tricky. This activity will help you identify the essential information that school staff, grandparents, babysitters, or activity leaders may need to keep your child safe, decide how much detail to share, and plan clear, simple language your child can also use. The goal is to balance safety, clarity, and practicality for each caregiving situation.

Decide Your Approach

List caregivers outside the home that you will or won't share information about treatment with:

☐ Yes ☐ No ☐ Not sure yet

__________________ __________________ __________________

__________________ __________________ __________________

__________________ __________________ __________________

If Yes, Why?

☐ They will be caring for the child during dosing time

☐ Rest period overlaps with school/activity hours

☐ Activity restrictions (gym, recess) are needed

☐ Symptoms may need monitoring while in others' care

☐ Other: __________________

Key Messages (Keep It Simple)

Fill in the information you want others to clearly understand:

☐ My child *is still allergic to:* _________________________________

☐ Safety precautions that must remain in place: ___________________________

☐ During treatment, my child: _________________________________

☐ Temporary accommodations needed: ___________________________

Treatment Communication Practice

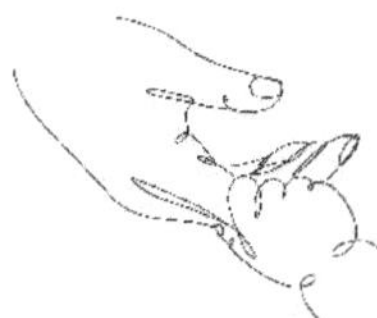 Children often want to share their progress, but others may not understand what their treatment really means. This activity helps your child practice clear, simple, and accurate ways to talk about their treatment with friends, teachers, or other caregivers so they can feel confident while keeping themselves safe.

Help your child practice a simple, clear, age-appropriate ways to talk about their treatment:

Preschool (Under 5)

- "I have a food allergy, and my doctor is helping me to be safer."

- "I still don't eat (allergen)" or "I still don't share food with friends."

- "Sometimes I need a quiet break after my dose."

Elementary (5–10 years)

- "I have an allergy, but my doctor is helping me eat a little bit safely."

- "I still need to avoid this food unless a grown-up says it's okay."

- "After I take it, I need to stay calm for a little while."

Upper Elementary (9–11 years)

- "I have a food allergy, and my treatment is helping me to safely eat small amounts."

- "I still follow all the safety rules, like reading labels and not sharing my food."

- "Sometimes I need to sit quietly for a few minutes after my dose."

Adolescent (12 and up)

- "I have a food allergy and am doing a treatment that lets me safely eat very small amounts with my doctor's supervision."

- "I'm still allergic and need to follow all the usual safety rules at school and with friends."

- "I may have to avoid activity for a while after taking my dose."

Part VI:
Staying the Course

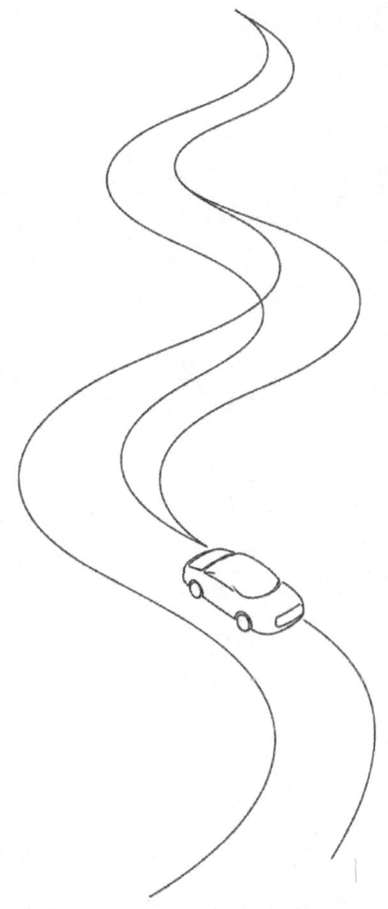

You can't go back and change the beginning,
but you can start where you are and change the ending.

— C.S. Lewis

Chapter 11:
Middle of the Road

Early Days of OIT: Finding a Rhythm

After the bumpy start, our early days of OIT gradually became easier. I had correctly anticipated that the biggest challenge would be the required rest period after dosing. Keeping three boys aged six and under calm for two hours every day was no small feat.

At first, we dosed at lunchtime so the rest period could overlap with the two youngest boys' naps. Unfortunately, they both stopped napping much younger than I had expected. My oldest had napped daily until after five, and I realized I'd been holding unrealistic expectations for the younger two. As with so many aspects of parenting young children, just when I felt we were settling into a rhythm, something shifted.

We continued dosing mid-day and eventually landed on a compromise: one hour of quiet time in their rooms (thank goodness for Legos), followed by an hour of television. The younger kids almost certainly watched more TV than I would have preferred at their ages, but it could have been worse. One thing that helped tremendously was that my son was perfectly happy eating a sunbutter-and-jelly sandwich every single day. Removing uncertainty and power struggles around food made the process feel much more manageable.

For a while, I was still nervous during the rest period, especially on days when keeping him calm felt harder. I came up with a reminder to ground myself: *I'd rather be nervous for two hours a day while we're in treatment than nervous all the time for the rest of his life.* That isn't to suggest that anyone *should* feel nervous all the time, but after the stretch of mystery and severe reactions we had endured, danger had felt omnipresent. This framing helped me tolerate the anxiety while staying committed to the process. My son didn't seem nervous at all. I think his doctor had made him feel so comfortable and confident that he simply enjoyed his Kool-Aid and the quiet time afterward.

At times, I struggled with feeling like I was constantly checking for signs of illness, monitoring his body, and deciding whether it was safe to dose. Early on, I wasn't comfortable leaving him with anyone else during dosing or the rest period. Over time, though, it became just another part of our daily routine. The family rhythm adjusted around it, and I began to feel a sense of trust in the treatment and his body's ability to adapt.

The Rhythm of Appointments and the Road

The routine of appointments was both difficult and wonderful. We developed our own system early on: packing his sunflower butter-and-jelly sandwich so he'd have a substantial lunch before his updose, and making pizza the night before so he could eat it cold on our long drive home. Establishing this routine helped us avoid unnecessary stops, saving both time and money. I felt fortunate to have a child who was a great eater yet found comfort in predictable food choices.

Car sickness added another layer of complexity. In the beginning, it was hard to tell whether nausea meant he was unwell and shouldn't dose, or if it was simply motion-related. Over time, we learned his patterns. Eventually, we waited until after he got sick before having him eat, so he'd still have food in his stomach for the updose. All the usual strategies helped: motion sickness bands, sitting in the middle seat, opening the windows for cool air, and making occasional stops.

Despite the nausea, those long drives became unexpectedly meaningful. We listened to music together, discovered podcasts we loved, devoured audiobooks, and bonded deeply during those hours on the road.

One of the most memorable days came after an appointment when my son was cleared for cross-contact, which meant he could now eat foods made in shared facilities or on shared equipment. On the drive home we saw seven rainbows, including one breathtaking, full double rainbow. We still talk about "rainbow day," remembering that time together with fondness and gratitude.

In It For the Long Haul

By the time you reach this stage of immunotherapy, so much has already been decided. You've gathered information, weighed options, and stepped into treatment. It may seem like the hardest part should be behind you, but it takes a different kind of work to maintain the treatment long-term.

It is normal to become exhausted or burnt out from the dedication immunotherapy treatments require. Children who are struggling with the routine or feeling anxious about their dosing rarely say, *"I'm overwhelmed by this treatment,"* or *"I feel anxious about this routine."* Even older children and adults may not have the language, insight, or comfort to express that directly.

Most of us, but especially children, communicate the internal world through behavior. During immunotherapy, when their bodies, routines, and sense of safety are being stretched, their behaviors can shift in ways that are easy to miss or misinterpret.

Here are some behaviors that might indicate that a child, teen, or adult is struggling with treatment:

Anger or Irritability
Big reactions that seem out of proportion or frustration that spills over into unrelated situations can reflect a nervous system that is on high alert, what we often call a fight-or-flight response. The treatment may not be named as the cause, but the body is carrying the load.

Difficulty Sleeping
Make note of trouble falling asleep, staying asleep, waking early, restless sleep, or increased nightmares. Sleep disruptions are one of the most common indicators of anxiety or overwhelm.

Defiance or Resistance
What can look like pushing back or being defiant may actually be an attempt to regain a sense of control.

When something feels unpredictable or outside of our control, it is natural to try to assert control wherever we can.

Emotional Outbursts
Seeming calm one moment and then suddenly "exploding" over something small or unrelated often reflects emotions that have been building under the surface and are finding a way out.

Difficulty Focusing
Trouble paying attention, seeming distracted, or "in their own world" can sometimes signal stress, not attention difficulties. Anxiety can pull attention inward, making it hard to stay present.

Avoidance
Hesitation or refusal around anything related to treatment or even things that feel indirectly connected (appointments, routines, conversations) is also noteworthy. Avoidance is a natural attempt to reduce discomfort, even if it limits coping over time.

Increased Negativity
More negative thinking, expecting the worst, or focusing on what could go wrong. This can function as a protective strategy. Anticipating something bad can help it feel less surprising or painful.

Overplanning or Needing Control
A strong desire to predict, plan, or control situations (even unrelated ones). This is another way to try to create a sense of safety and predictability when something feels uncertain.

What This Means (and What It Doesn't)

Changes in mood, behavior, or internal experience are not signs that you or your child are "failing" treatment. They are signals that the nervous system is working hard to process something that is both physically and emotionally complex and demanding.

If you are a parent, this may show up in your child's behavior. If you are a teen or adult in treatment, this may show up in your thoughts, your body, or your reactions to everyday situations. Either way, these responses are not problems to eliminate. They are information to understand.

What Can Help
Start with curiosity. If you are a parent, gently explore what you're noticing in your child without assuming or pushing for clear answers. Many children won't be able to directly connect what they're feeling to treatment, but they can still benefit from feeling seen, supported, and not "in trouble" for how they're reacting.

If you are a teen or adult, this may look like slowing down and noticing your own patterns with compassion. You might ask yourself questions without needing immediate answers. *What has been feeling harder lately? What feels different in my body or my reactions?*

One of the most powerful tools at any age is a sense of control. For parents, this means offering choice wherever possible, even if the treatment routine itself isn't flexible. Small decisions like what to wear, what to eat, small aspects of daily routines, or how to spend free time can return a sense of control.

For teens and adults, this may look like identifying where you *do* have agency: how you prepare, how you structure your day, and how you care for yourself before and after dosing. These moments of choice help restore balance when other parts of the experience feel less flexible or predictable.

If these reactions or patterns feel persistent, overwhelming, or difficult to navigate, seeking therapeutic support can be incredibly helpful, not because something is "wrong," but because everyone deserves space to process this experience with guidance and support.

Treatment Check-In Worksheet

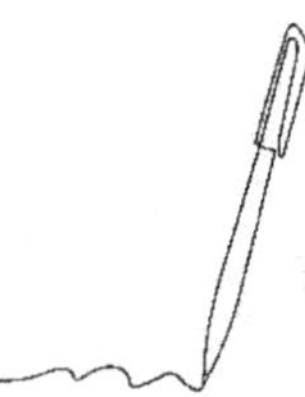

Use this worksheet anytime during treatment to reflect on your thoughts and feelings so far. It can be helpful when questions arise, new milestones happen, or when you notice setbacks, changes, or progress.

You can also use these prompts to start a discussion with your child. Choose one to three questions at a time depending on their age, and encourage them to write, draw, or say aloud their thoughts, feelings, and questions while you make notes. These may also be helpful to discuss while taking a walk, working on a craft, or having a snack together rather than as a more structured conversation.

Reflect on the Current Experience

- How are things going with treatment right now?
- Have there been any changes in symptoms, reactions, or side effects?
- Are there any challenges or setbacks?
- Have there been any successes, milestones, or progress to celebrate?

____
____
____
____
____

Explore Thoughts and Feelings

- How do I feel about the treatment right now?
- Am I worried about anything?
- Is there anything confusing or unclear?
- What parts feel easy or comforting?

____
____
____
____
____

Problem-Solving and Planning

- What can I do at home to support comfort and safety?
- Are there adjustments I should make to routines, dosing, or monitoring?
- Are there strategies to make treatment easier or more predictable?

____

____

____

____

____

Next Steps & Follow-Up

- What is the first thing I should do after completing this check-in?
- Who will help with any questions or concerns?
- When should I revisit this worksheet again?

____

____

____

____

____

Questions For My Care Team

____

____

____

____

____

Allergy Adventure Check-In

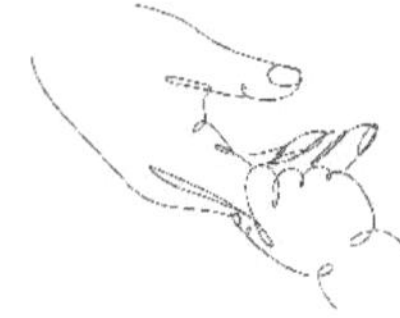

This worksheet turns immunotherapy progress into an adventure your child is actively part of. It helps them reflect on challenges, successes, and questions. Use this page with your progress map, or create your own version of this to match the theme you chose for your child's sticker/motivation chart.

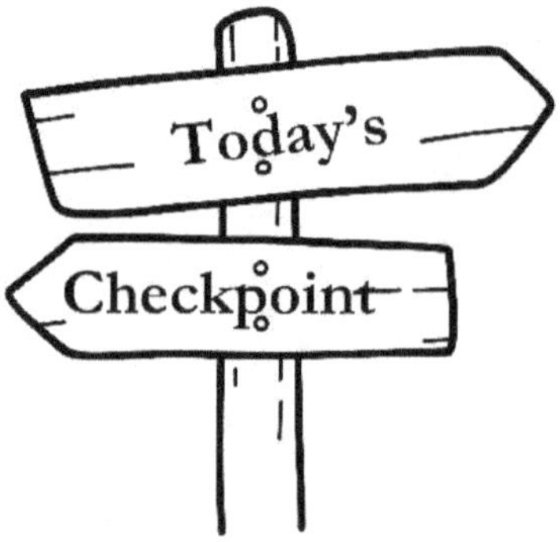

Today's
Checkpoint

Today I:

Easiest part:

Hardest part:

Feelings Compass"

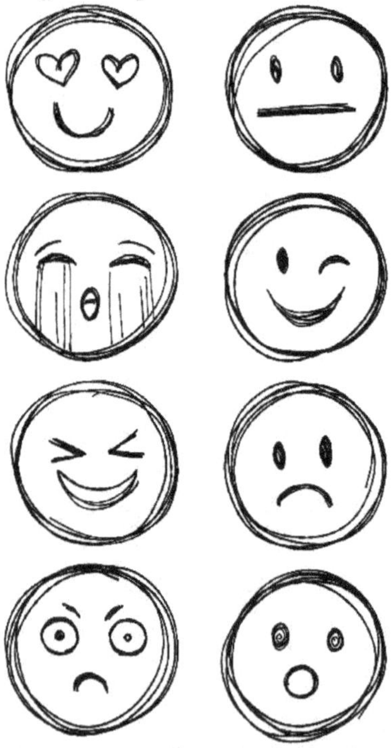

Thoughts and Questions:

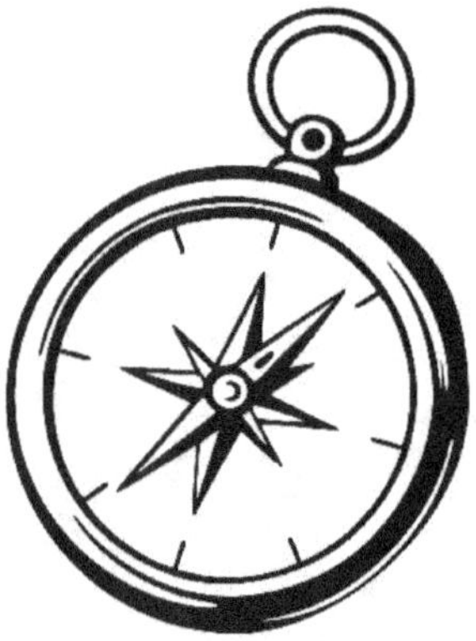

Future plan:

Transitioning to Whole Food Doses

Some of the most defining moments in our immunotherapy journey didn't happen in the doctor's office. They happened in the quiet, ordinary spaces where the weight of what we were doing seemed to suddenly catch up with me and register in the real world. One of those moments was in the middle of a grocery store aisle, standing in front of shelves lined with bags of peanuts.

We had reached the point where it was time to transition from liquid doses to real pieces of peanut. Logically, I knew my son had already been safely consuming peanut in liquid form. I trusted the process and I trusted our doctor. And yet, standing there trying to decide which bag to buy, I felt completely overwhelmed.

A small bag? A large one? His doses were tiny, but we would need a lot over time. I stood there quietly crying, staring at options that felt far heavier than they should have. Eventually, I picked up the largest bulk bag I could find and placed it in the cart. They went stale before we used them all. But in that moment, choosing that bag felt like a commitment to fully step into this next phase of the journey, and an act of defiance against the food that had terrorized us.

The transition to whole food doses marked a shift in more ways than one. Practically, things became easier. We no longer had to rely on compounded mixtures or frequent trips just to pick up the next dose even if we were sick and unable to updose. Those beginning months of treatment had been exhausting, but emotionally, this transition felt almost like starting over.

In my clinical work, I see this often. When a treatment moves from something diluted and medicalized into something that is visibly and obviously the allergen itself, it can bring everything back to the surface. For us, squirting a tiny amount of liquid into his mouth had felt contained, controlled, and almost separate from the food itself. Watching him pick up a piece of peanut and eat it was entirely different.

We talked about it many times beforehand. I explained that the liquid doses were like medicine, slowly and safely teaching his body that peanuts were not an enemy. As we approached this milestone, I reminded him that the medicine had done its job, and that the doctor knew when his body was ready for more.

Still, when the moment came, he hesitated.

At his first whole-food dose in the office, he paused before even picking up the peanut. I held my breath, unsure whether he would follow through. Part of me was afraid he would refuse. Another part of me felt overwhelmed with awe. After all the time, energy, fear, and effort we had poured into this process, we were finally here.

Our doctor handled the moment perfectly. There was no over-explaining, no amplifying the fear. Just a simple acknowledgment: it's normal to feel hesitant, and you're safe. Then a gentle redirection: I wonder if you'll like the taste.

He didn't.

I can still picture his tiny fingers holding that piece of peanut: the slight wince as he put it in his mouth, the way he wiped his hands quickly, chewed slowly, and then shrugged as if nothing monumental had just happened.

That moment marked a turning point, not because it erased the past or guaranteed an easy road ahead, but because something that once felt dangerous and impossible was now safe and commonplace.

Exploring Dosing Options

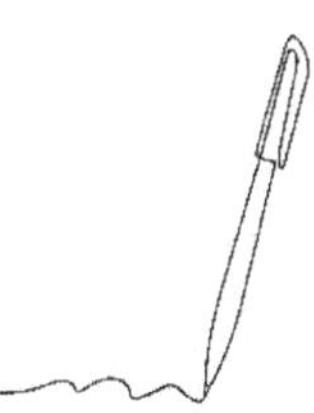

For many people with food allergies, the idea of eating something they are not used to and were told was dangerous is scary. If they have a history of reactions, they may associate that food with feeling very sick, and sometimes the sight or even smell of it can feel overwhelming. Resistance, smell or texture issues, and strong preferences are common while undergoing immunotherapy and are completely normal.

This section is designed to give strategies and different forms of each of the top 9 allergens if you or your child are having trouble tolerating them. Options may include changing the texture, incorporating small amounts into recipes, or pairing the allergen with a preferred food.

Important: Everyone's treatment plan is individualized and dosing must be very precise. *Always check with your allergist before:*

- Eating your allergen in a different form than what you were provided/instructed
- Cooking, baking, or freezing the allergen
- Combining the allergen with other ingredients
- Altering the dose form (e.g., powder, paste, whole food)

Some allergens respond differently to heat, freezing, or processing, and certain immunotherapy protocols and providers specifically advise against certain preparations. In some cases, modifying the allergen without medical guidance can affect both safety and treatment effectiveness.

Many focus on hiding the taste in chocolate, candy, or sweet baked goods. While this may work for some, many say that this only makes the taste of the allergen stand out more. As a general rule, if sweet hasn't worked, try savory. This seems to be particularly true for peanuts, tree nuts, and sesame.

Use this list as a guide and brainstorming tool, not a prescription or medical advice. If your provider has approved a new form of the food or approach to dosing, you will need to work closely with them to determine how to get the exact amount of allergen into each dose. Carefully track what works and doesn't work for you and your child, and bring notes to your allergist to adjust the plan as needed.

Think of this like picking different lanes on the road. All routes lead to the same destination, but some need careful permission from the guide (your allergist) before proceeding.

Dosing Alternative Ideas for the Top 9 Allergens

REMEMBER: DO NOT MAKE ANY CHANGES TO YOUR DOSING ROUTINE WITHOUT YOUR DOCTOR'S APPROVAL

Peanuts/Tree nuts* Whole nuts: chopped/ground, mix in trail mix with safe chocolate chips/raisins/candy. This works especially well if the child is dosing multiple nuts. Bake into cookies/muffins. Add to smoothies. Grind and mix into soft foods like applesauce, yogurt, chocolate syrup, pudding. Dip in chocolate and chill/freeze (many report this decreases the flavor significantly). If your child can swallow pills, ask your doctor if you can chop finely and place into empty capsules.
-Nut butters: spread on crackers, dip for pretzels or fruit
-Nut powders: mix into liquids, smoothies, bake/cook
-Nut milks: Sometimes used but often do not contain enough of the allergen's protein needed for dosing. If approved by your doctor, can be mixed with syrups or powders for chocolate/strawberry/etc. Dilute with milk of choice if necessary
-Nut puffs: (Bamba, Mighty Me Mission puffs)

Milk**: Add to cereal, hot chocolate, dip/crumble cookies into it. Powdered milk mixed into sauces, smoothies, spreads. Yogurt or cheese as a dip or topping.

Egg**: Whole cooked egg (scrambled, hard-boiled), egg powder mixed into pancakes, muffins, sauces, baked egg in recipes

Wheat: Bread or toast spread with any toppings (safe butter, jam, peanut/nut butters, Nutella), pasta combined with sauce of preference, flour/baking mixes

Soy: Soy milk in smoothies or with cereal, tofu blend into recipes (soups, stir-fries), soy protein powder mixed into sauces, spreads, smoothies

Fish/Shellfish*: Cooked fish flakes with various spices, mixed with tolerated foods like rice, vegetables, meat, pureed fish/shellfish incorporated into soups and dips, canned fish

Sesame: tahini, sesame seeds (usually not given whole because the seed hull prevents digestion and it passes whole through the body), sesame paste, sesame flour, hummus

*Allergens (peanuts/tree nuts, fish/shellfish) that have similar form/texture are combined here to reduce redundancy. Carefully check with your provider that you use the correct form of the correct nut needed for your treatment protocol. For example, sometimes changing from a raw form to a roasted form of a tree nut can impact treatment.

**Be especially careful to clarify with your doctor which forms of the allergen are acceptable. The immunotherapy process is different from working your way up the egg/milk ladders.

Allergy Dose Tracking Worksheet

Instructions: Use one worksheet per allergen to track ideas, attempts, and preferences. Print extra copies as needed. Consider allowing your child to use stickers or draw smiley/frowny faces beside different options.

Allergen: ____

Date	Dose Form	Doctor Approved?	Notes (child's preference, ease of prep/eating, etc.)

Chapter 12:
Turbulence

The Bumps in Our Road

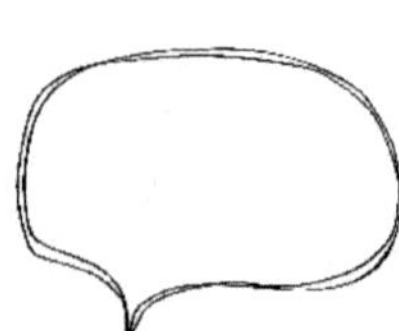

Given my son's history of extreme sensitivity and unpredictable, statistically unlikely reactions, I was certain we would encounter significant challenges during his build-up phase. To my surprise, he moved through it with remarkable steadiness. In the early days, I held my breath waiting for something to go wrong, but it didn't.

I'd become mostly comfortable with our dosing routine by the time my son experienced a reaction. It reminded us that even on a well-mapped road, there can still be unexpected turns. It was an ordinary day. He had completed his dose and finished his two-hour rest period without issue. About two hours and fifteen minutes later, he came downstairs and started playing a video game.

Then, he began to cough. At first, it was subtle, but it escalated quickly. For a moment, I hesitated and stood there in disbelief. His anaphylactic reaction to the peanut patch years earlier had presented primarily as coughing, something that had confused us both at the time. Because of that experience, we recognized the pattern much more quickly now. This time, we didn't stay stuck in uncertainty.

My son was hesitant to use his epinephrine, insisting he was fine even though he clearly wasn't. (He remembers this day well and how much he just wanted to keep playing his video game.) I calmly pulled out the printed instructions from his allergist, and pointed to the exact criteria that applied to what he was experiencing. Seeing it in writing helped him acknowledge what needed to be done.

With some encouragement, he decided to administer the epinephrine himself for the first time. Almost immediately, the coughing subsided and his irritated skin calmed down. We called the ambulance, packed a bag, and when the paramedics arrived, we were ready. He was already feeling better, but was glad to go to the hospital for some reassurance.

Several things changed after that experience. His allergist recommended extending his rest period to two and a half hours moving forward. We kept the printed instructions in his epi pouch, because we realized that looking at them and pointing to the symptoms on the page made it very clear what to do. Most important, his confidence grew exponentially. Instead of fearing his epinephrine, he had a new respect and appreciation for it and his ability to use it if needed. He was proud of himself for doing something brave.

Although I had worried that this would happen, the experience was much different than I thought it would be. This reaction didn't feel chaotic and confusing like accidental exposures had in the past. It happened within a known window of caution, where we were home monitoring him and equipped to respond. There was no mystery, no delayed realization, no lingering questions or self-blame about what mistake I'd made or figuring out if/how he'd accidentally been exposed to an allergen.

This is one of the paradoxes of immunotherapy that can be hard to grasp from the outside: The idea of intentionally introducing allergens and the possibility of reactions can feel terrifying in theory.

In practice, there can be something profoundly regulating about having a defined area of time in which to pay careful attention, and seeing the worry outside that boundary shrink.

Reactions and Anaphylaxis in OIT: What Families Should Know

 When families consider oral immunotherapy (OIT), a wide range of emotions swirl around the possibility of reactions and anaphylaxis. Adverse reactions are observed in most patients undergoing OIT, with mild symptoms occurring more often, and with severe reactions being less common (Nachshon et al., 2021).

Research indicates that between 10% to 20% of participants undergoing oral immunotherapy (OIT) require epinephrine at some point during the desensitization process (Romantsik et al., 2018; Yeung et al., 2012). While these events do occur, remember that patients are dosing daily, so reactions represent a very small proportion of total exposures to the allergens (Wasserman et al., 2014). It is also important to understand that the vast majority of these occur during the updosing phase of treatment, and are not typically an ongoing problem once the maintenance phase is reached (Vickery et al., 2018).

The above statistics must be interpreted carefully. Protocols differ across clinics, statistics vary by allergens, and co-factors such as illness, exercise, stress, or missed meals can increase the likelihood of reactions. Every clinician will have their own protocol, thresholds, and guidelines for managing reactions during OIT. These are individualized and often adjusted over time based on response patterns. Open communication with your allergist about history, symptoms, and daily realities increases both safety and trust. Clarity and confidence around when to use epinephrine, how to interpret symptoms, and when to seek urgent care helps patients and families feel supported and empowered rather than alone in the process.

Bringing Instructions Into the Real World
One practical recommendation is to keep a printed copy of your action plan and emergency instructions wherever dosing takes place. Even if this information is available electronically, having it physically accessible during moments of stress can be grounding and clarifying.

When you are calm, decisions about whether to use epinephrine may feel straightforward. In the middle of an unexpected reaction, however, the body's threat response can narrow attention and make recall more difficult. Having a written plan serves as an external guide, helping you respond based on clear instructions rather than fear alone.

From a psychological perspective, this reduces cognitive load and supports more regulated decision-making under stress. External decision aids in medical settings have been shown to improve adherence and reduce anxiety by providing clear, structured guidance during high-pressure situations (Ryan & Hill, 2024).

What This Means for You
OIT is a process with both risks and benefits. Mild symptoms are common and often manageable. Severe reactions, including anaphylaxis, do occur but are relatively uncommon when treatment protocols are followed and epinephrine is used appropriately.

This section is not meant to minimize the reality of anaphylaxis. Rather, it places it in context: a known but manageable possibility within a structured and closely monitored treatment plan. With preparation, support, and clear communication, families can navigate reactions with greater confidence and care.

Ongoing Assessment for Trauma

 If you find yourself or your child reacting strongly after an unexpected reaction or difficult experience, it may be helpful to consider whether this might be a trauma response. When something frightening or unpredictable happens in the body, especially in the context of food allergies, the nervous system can hold onto that experience in a way that continues to influence how safe things feel moving forward.

You may notice increased fear, hesitation, physical symptoms, or a loss of trust in a process that previously felt manageable. If that happens, it does not mean you have done anything wrong or that treatment is no longer an option. It may mean that your nervous system needs time, support, and space to process what happened before continuing. You can return to the chapter of this book on trauma for a deeper understanding of this, and consider whether additional support may be helpful as you decide how to move forward.

Anaphylaxis Debrief

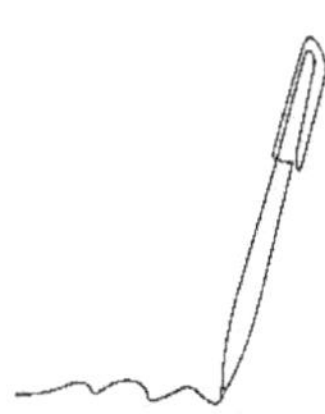

Experiencing an anaphylactic reaction during OIT can be intense. It's normal to experience lingering stress, worry, or heightened vigilance. Reflecting on the experience helps to process what happened, identify what went well, and strengthen confidence for future dosing. Hopefully you never need this page, but if you do, I hope it helps you feel more grounded and less alone after a scary experience.

This is a reflection and integration activity. It is not a replacement for trauma therapy. If you are already working with a therapist, consider reviewing this experience together. If distress feels intense, persistent, or worsening over time, consulting a mental health professional may be supportive. Always use your judgment and consult your allergist as needed.

Even if you feel calm or fine, completing this worksheet can help your nervous system "download" the experience and reinforce the sense of safety and preparedness for the future.

Immediate Practical Recovery

Note what might be helpful for you:

☐ Hydration   ☐ Food (once cleared to eat)   ☐ Rest or reduced demands

☐ Quiet/familiar environment ☐ Check-in with medical provider ☐ Written follow-up guidance

☐ Trusted company   ☐ A distracting activity/outing   ☐ Other:

____

____

Reflect on the Reaction:

Symptoms (coughing, hives, swelling, throat tightness, timing, location)

____

____

Actions Taken (epinephrine administered, steps on plan that were followed, other steps taken)

____

____

What went well or didn't go well (epinephrine administered quickly, child self-administered, stayed calm enough to follow the plan)

____

____

Physical and Emotional Debrief

How my body felt during and after

☐ Shaking or trembling ☐ Fatigue ☐ Emotional sensitivity

☐ Heightened alertness or worry ☐ Headache or soreness ☐ Difficulty sleeping

☐ Heart rate changes ☐ Muscle tension ☐ Nausea

☐ Other:

____

____

Emotional reactions (Remember, strong emotions often surface later, not during the emergency)

☐ Relief ☐ Fear ☐ Guilt ☐ Anger

☐ Sadness ☐ Gratitude ☐ Exhaustion ☐ Proud

☐ Worried ☐ In Shock ☐ Helpless ☐ Disoriented

☐ Other:

____

____

Complete this sentence and repeat it to yourself:

"It makes sense that I feel _______________________________ after this experience."

Reassuring thoughts and self-talk

☐ I did everything right ☐ It's all okay now ☐ We handled this together

☐ The medicine did its job ☐ I can handle this feeling ☐ I will get through this

☐ Other:

____

____

Communication & Support

Who I can debrief with (Partner, friend, doctor, other family, OIT staff)

____

____

What I want to share (What to get off your chest? What might be helpful for them to know/do?)

____

____

Repair and Reassurance

For yourself: What would you say to a close friend who went through this?

____

____

Now offer that same statement to yourself.

For your child (if applicable): What message(s) do you want them to internalize after this experience?

☐ Your body needed help, and we gave it. ☐ You did not do anything wrong.

☐ We were prepared and we knew what to do. ☐ It's over now.

☐ I'm right here. I'm not going anywhere. ☐ We can get through anything together.

Write your own:

____

____

Planning Ahead

Next steps for dosing (Refill epi, review action plan, adjust rest periods, document the incident, schedule follow-up with allergist)

____

____

Calming or grounding activity (Mindful breathing, walk, music, journaling, cuddling a pet)

____

____

Takeaways

Has this experience taught you anything? Strengthened your confidence? Given you something to remember moving forward?

____

____

Recovery is not about erasing fear but about helping your system learn that you can move through hard moments and come out the other side.

Calming and Connecting After A Reaction

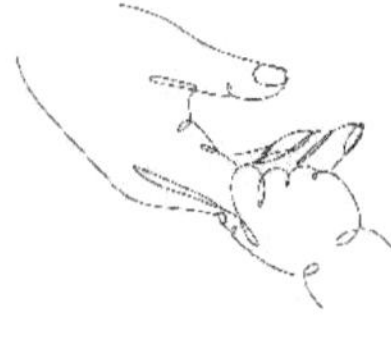 Use this as a guide to help your child process the incident, validate their feelings, and reinforce trust in epinephrine and safety moving forward with treatment. Remember this activity is about connection and emotional expression, not correction. Invite your child to share, but don't force them.

Materials:

- Paper and markers or crayons
- Puppets, stuffed animals, or action figures
- Stickers, stamps (optional)

Reminder:

Mirror your child's language throughout this activity, and anytime afterward when discussing the topic. If they call the reaction "the hospital day," continue to call it that until their language shifts.

Tell the Story

Invite your child to draw, act out, or tell the story of what happened in their own words. Use puppets or stuffed animals, a toy doctor kit, and any other items around the home if helpful.

- Encourage them to show:
    - What the body felt like
    - What actions were taken
    - What helped (medications, comfort measures)
    - Who helped them

Emotion Mapping

- Ask the child how they would show the different emotions and sensations they experienced on paper or using toys. Help them give words to the emotions and validate these feelings.

What Went Well

- Discuss how epinephrine worked to stop the reaction, and what helpers played a role
- Ask your child to draw or write a "thank you" note to their epinephrine (it could be a simple sentence, drawing, or sticker), or anyone who helped them during and after the reaction
- Ask the child to identify 1–2 things that helped them feel safer or comforted them (focus on specific details or sensory experiences of safety)
- Celebrate these successes with a small ritual (high five, sticker, or hug)

Use simple, reassuring language

- "Your body needed help, and we helped it."
- "The medicine worked."
- "You did not do anything wrong."
- "Grownups and doctors know how to help."

Choose a comforting activity:

- Favorite show
- Going for a walk or playing outside
- Drawing, coloring, or painting
- Music or reading together
- Provide physical

Note for caregivers:

If your child shows ongoing distress such as nightmares or sleep difficulties, avoidance of dosing or other regular activities, significant changes in eating, or persistent fear or other big emotions, consider checking in with a pediatric mental health professional. This activity supports processing but does not replace therapy.

Notes about your child's comments and responses

____
____
____
____
____
____
____

Worksheet: Preparing to Dose Again After a Reaction

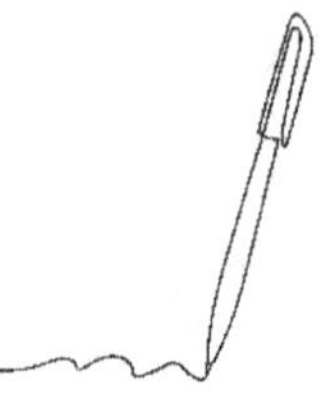

This worksheet helps you process your feelings, track your body's responses, and build confidence for safely returning to dosing after a reaction. *It is only recommended if you are experiencing resistance or anxiety about dosing again following the reaction.* Please refer to the recommendations on recognizing trauma and consider whether additional support would be helpful.

Reflect on the Reaction

- What sensations of the reaction are coming back to me now?
- What steps were effective in responding to that reaction?
- How did the plan/medication help stop the reaction?

____

____

____

____

Body Scan

- What sensations am I noticing now when I think about dosing again?
  (e.g., increased heart rate, tightness, tension, stomach butterflies, trembling, racing thoughts, sweaty)
- Rate intensity from 0–10

____

____

____

____

Thoughts & Feelings

- What worries or fears come up about dosing again?
- What information and evidence can remind me that I am prepared and safe?

____

____

____

____

Plan & Support

- What steps will I take to prepare for dosing?
  (e.g., review action plan, set up space, have calming activity ready, involve a trusted person)
- Who and what can support me during dosing?

____

____

____

____

Calm & Grounding

- Identify a grounding item or activity to use before, during, or after dosing:
  (favorite object, music, breath exercise, short movement, mantra)

____

____

____

____

Reflection After Dosing

- How did my body respond?
- How did I handle my emotions?
- What did I learn about myself, my child, or my confidence in the plan?

____

____

____

____

____

____

____

Guide for Considering Additional Support After a Reaction

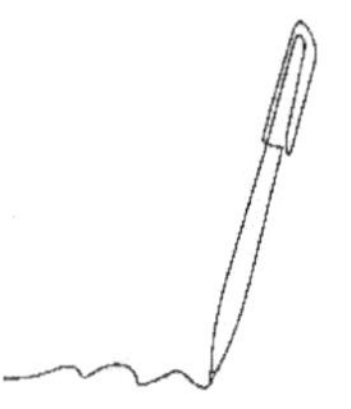

Most patients and families recover well after an allergic reaction with rest, support and medical follow-up. However, sometimes reactions can leave lingering stress or trauma-like symptoms.

Signs that additional mental health support may be helpful include:

For Parents/Teens/Adults:

- ☐ Difficulty sleeping or recurring nightmares about dosing or reactions
- ☐ Excessive sleep, can't get out of bed or get going
- ☐ Persistent anxiety that interferes with daily life or dosing
- ☐ Hypervigilance or excessive avoidance of safe situations
- ☐ Social withdrawal, avoiding work/school or friends
- ☐ Intrusive thoughts about the reaction
- ☐ Feeling emotionally numb, detached, or easily startled
- ☐ Changes in appetite, weight, or clothing fit

For Children:

- ☐ Repeated fears about dosing or any daily/routine activities
- ☐ Changes in appetite, weight, or clothing fit
- ☐ Regression in behavior or independence, clinginess
- ☐ Nightmares or difficulty sleeping
- ☐ Physical complaints (stomachaches, headaches), may or may not be linked to worry
- ☐ Withdrawal or clinginess beyond typical developmental behavior
- ☐ Avoiding school, activities, or events outside the home

Recommendations:

- ☐ Consult with a therapist if distress persists for more than 1–2 weeks or intensifies
- ☐ Consult your allergist if anxiety is interfering with dosing or routine care
- ☐ Normalizing feelings and validating emotions is helpful, but professional guidance ensures trauma symptoms are addressed early

Please remember: This workbook provides educational and reflective tools, but it is *not a replacement for therapy or medical care*. Always follow your allergist's guidance for dosing, accidental exposure reactions, epinephrine use, and OIT-related emergencies, and ask them for resources (therapists, local allergy advocacy group) if more support would be helpful.

Roll to Reset

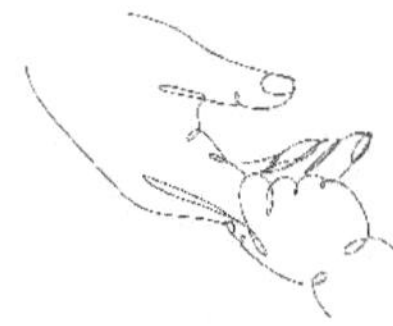 Big feelings can make our bodies feel busy, tense, or overwhelmed. The best way to reset is usually not to "fix" the feeling, but to help the body feel safe first. This game is a simple way to practice regulation together after any tough moment.

Kids and adults will take turns rolling the dice 3 times each. Each time you roll, you complete the activity listed by that number under that turn. Every number matches a different type of calming activity. Remember to engage in the activity with your child, not just ask them to roll and participate in the skills.

Roll	Activity	Turn 1	Turn 2	Turn 3
⚀	Breathing	Smell the dandelion, then blow out the seeds (3x)	Balloon belly breathing: hands on belly and slowly fill it up like a balloon (30 seconds)	Breathe in like a fierce dragon; blow the worry or stress away (3x)
⚁	Grounding	Hold something cold. Describe how it feels	Sip a cold or warm drink. Notice how it feels in your mouth and throat	Find something for each color of the rainbow in the space around you
⚂	Stretching	On your hands and knees, stretch like a sleepy cat	Make a rainbow with your arms, standing tall and reaching from one side to the other	Stand tall like a tree with your feet rooted to the ground. Reach your arms up like branches and sway
⚃	Moving	Shake your whole body for 15 seconds	30 second dance break to music of your choice	Walk around the room like your favorite animal for 30 seconds
⚄	Connecting	Choose a hug, hand hold, high five, or fist bump	Look into each other's eyes for 15 seconds (and try not to laugh!)	Say something you like about each other
⚅	Affirming	Say to each other or yourself in the mirror: "I've got this."	Say to each other or to yourself in the mirror: "We'll figure it out together."	Say to each other or to yourself in the mirror: "I can do hard things."

Chapter 13:
Course Correction

Evaluating a Treatment Path

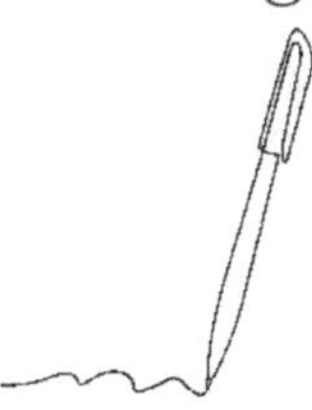

When bumps in the road happen, it is natural to have strong emotional reactions, second-guess our decisions, and to consider stopping. Pausing to reflect on decisions before moving forward with them can help to clarify our reasoning, lower emotional reactivity, and even improve outcomes.

What initially drew me to this treatment option? What was I hoping it would change?

____

____

What feels supportive about this treatment so far?

____

____

What feels heavy, overwhelming, or unsustainable?

____

____

How do I hope this treatment will affect me/my child?

____

____

What signs tell me it is working, progress is being made, or continuing could be a positive choice?

____

____

What signs indicate that I should consider pausing or pivoting?

____

____

When I imagine continuing this treatment for the time it will require, my body feels:

____

____

When I imagine stopping or changing course, my body feels:

____

____

The Slow Work of Feeling Safe Again

After my son transitioned to peanut pieces and eventually multiple peanuts and cashews, too, things began to gradually and quietly shift. Each successful dose built on the one before it. And as he adapted, I found myself changing too.

I stopped worrying about every surface the nuts had touched in the kitchen. I stopped washing my hands every time I handled them. I caught myself mid-wash and reminded myself, over and over: *he is eating this food safely*. But the emotional adjustment didn't happen all at once.

There were moments when I struggled internally, and he was completely fine. There were moments when he felt unsure, and I was steady. Somewhere in that overlap, I think each other's bravery carried us forward.

Another major shift came when we began incorporating foods with "may contain" or cross-contact labels. That shift from strict avoidance to intentional inclusion felt big in a different way. Seeing those words on a package and choosing to move forward anyway required a level of trust that gradually felt normal over time, not the day the doctor gave us the go-ahead for cross-contact.

One of my favorite memories from this phase was how we chose to celebrate, and I think it cemented the transition for us. We went to a popular local donut shop we had never tried before. We stood together in front of the case, taking in rows of colorful donut flavors we'd never tried.

He read the allergy sign carefully. He asked questions. He made his choice. Then he turned around and stood proudly as I took his picture with that sign, warning about the potential for cross-contact with his allergens. I continued taking way too many pictures while the rest of the family ate donuts for dinner.

What I came to understand, again and again, is that increased safety does not automatically create a sense of calm. Our nervous systems didn't update as quickly as the facts do. Confidence didn't come from a single moment or just because someone, even a doctor, told us it's safe. It built over time.

The first dose in the doctor's office felt overwhelming. The first time he ate it at home felt just as big. Then each time it was eaten safely, gradually and quietly in the background of repeated experiences, I found myself responding differently. Without quite realizing when it happened, I recognized that I was no longer watching in disbelief. My son was safely eating the food that had once sent him to the hospital in the ambulance, gasping for air.

When Safety Changes, But Your Nervous System Hasn't Caught Up Yet

One of the most disorienting parts of this journey is that progress might not *feel* like progress. You might expect that as safety increases, anxiety will decrease in equal measure. It makes sense to expect that once a food is introduced, cross-contact is cleared, or a dose is tolerated again and again, your body will finally exhale, but that's not always how it works.

The Nervous System Learns Through Repetition, Not Logic

From a psychological and neurobiological perspective, anxiety is a protective mechanism, not a flaw. When you or your child has experienced real risk, especially unpredictable or severe reactions, your brain and body adapt by becoming more vigilant. This is a protective process rooted in conditioning and threat detection. Even when the situation changes medically, that learning doesn't automatically update.

This is why, even well into treatment, eating a food that is now considered safe can still feel unsafe, seeing "may contain" on a label can still trigger a stress response, touching or being near a previously dangerous allergen can still feel activating, and letting go of routines that once kept you safe can still feel deeply uncomfortable. This is not irrational. This is your nervous system holding tightly to the ways it worked so hard to keep you safe.

Why Progress Can Feel Unsettling (Even When It's Positive)

One of the most important reasons progress can be distressing is *extinction learning*, the process by which the brain gradually "unlearns" a fear response when a previously threatening stimulus is repeatedly experienced without harm. This is the same mechanism underlying exposure-based therapies for anxiety. However, extinction learning is not immediate. It is gradual, requires consistent repetition, and is highly context-dependent. A single successful exposure is not enough for the brain to fully update its sense of safety. Confidence develops through many experiences over time (Craske et al., 2014).

At the same time, many of the *safety precautions* that once served an essential role begin to shift. The routines you developed, like carefully reading every label, avoiding certain environments, washing hands and surfaces, and tightly controlling food preparation, were not simply habits. They were strategies that helped you feel safe in an unpredictable context. As treatment progresses, letting go of these behaviors can feel unsettling even though they are no longer needed. Research in anxiety shows that safety behaviors are protective in the short term, but can become deeply reinforced over time, making them difficult to release even when the level of threat changes (Salkovskis, 1991).

In addition, many families experience an *identity shift* during this stage. Food allergy often becomes an integral part of how individuals see themselves and their roles within the family. You may have come to identify as the vigilant one, the prepared one, the advocate, or the person responsible for keeping everyone safe. As these roles begin to change, it can lead to a sense of disorientation. Even positive identity shifts can feel destabilizing because they require integrating a new way of being with an old one that was shaped by years of lived experience.

Another layer that often emerges is *grief*, which can coexist alongside progress. This can be surprising and, at times, confusing. Families may find themselves grieving the years spent in fear, the energy required to reach this point, or the experiences that felt out of reach during earlier stages of the journey. There may also be a growing awareness of just how much was carried along the way.

Finally, even as objective risk decreases, the brain continues to hold onto memories of *worst-case scenario* thinking. This is particularly true in food allergy life, where the consequences of reactions can be severe. Research consistently shows that perceived health risk, not just actual risk, plays a significant role in quality of life (Li et al., 2020). In other words, how dangerous something feels can influence daily functioning just as much as the statistical likelihood of harm.

These processes help explain why this phase of immunotherapy can feel emotionally complex. Understanding these patterns can make it easier to approach this stage with compassion, patience, and realistic expectations.

Confidence Comes From Doing, Not Knowing

Confidence is not something you think your way into. It is experienced incrementally as we measure and eat the dose over and over again. You are not behind if you're not fully relaxed yet. You are in the process of adjusting.

What Helps the Adjustment Process

While time and repetition are central, there are ways to support this transition:

- Name what's happening ("My body is still catching up")

- Move gradually rather than forcing sudden leaps

- Stay connected to medical guidance while allowing emotional processing

- Practice regulation strategies alongside exposure (breathing, grounding, pacing)

- Acknowledge both progress and discomfort at the same time

Mapping Your Milestones

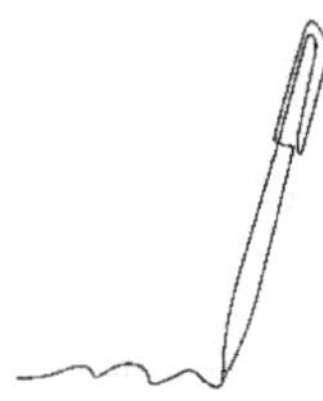

In treatment, progress is often measured in dose increases, foods added, reactions avoided. But the inner mental/emotional shifts don't always happen at the same pace as the measurable medical progress.

This activity helps you track your *emotional progress*. By mapping your milestones you can begin to see how your comfort, confidence, and sense of safety evolve over time. As you move through treatment (or even as you reflect back), use this page to document the meaningful milestones. These can be small or significant moments where something once felt hard, scary, or uncertain, and you got through it.

This can help you to both celebrate and acknowledge progress mid-journey, looking back and realizing how difficult something might have been in the past and is no longer quite so challenging. You can complete this page over time, adding new milestones or experiences as you reach them.

1. First time I... ____

(example: ate a "may contain" food, dosed without anxiety, traveled with my medication, etc.)

How I felt before: ____
How I felt after: ____
What helped me get through it: ____

2. First time I... ____

How I felt before: ____
How I felt after: ____
What helped me get through it: ____

3. First time I... ____

How I felt before: ____
How I felt after: ____
What helped me get through it: ____

4. First time I... ____

How I felt before: ____
How I felt after: ____
What helped me get through it: ____

5. First time I… ___________________________________

How I felt before: ___________________________________
How I felt after: ___________________________________
What helped me get through it: ___________________________________

6. First time I… ___________________________________

How I felt before: ___________________________________
How I felt after: ___________________________________
What helped me get through it: ___________________________________

7. First time I… ___________________________________

How I felt before: ___________________________________
How I felt after: ___________________________________
What helped me get through it: ___________________________________

Reflection

Looking back at these moments:

What patterns do you notice in how your confidence has grown?

____
____

Are there things that once felt impossible that now feel manageable, or even routine?

____
____

What does this tell you about your capacity to adapt, even when it feels hard?

____
____

Progress isn't just about what your body can tolerate.
It's also about what your mind learns it can trust.

My Confidence Ladder

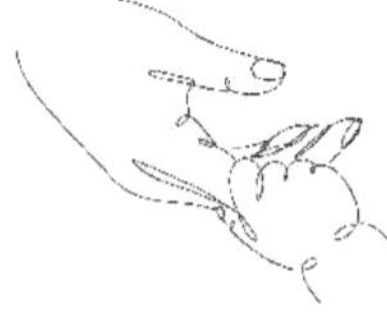

Seeing how far you've already climbed

This activity helps your child recognize their progress during treatment. Kids and adults tend to focus on what still feels hard, but this activity helps us acknowledge together what they've already done, step by step.

Imagine your progress like climbing a ladder. Each step you take, whether big or small, helps you move higher. Let's fill in your ladder together!

My Goal (Top of the Ladder)
What is your biggest reason for doing
immunotherapy?
(Feeling safe eating my foods,
being able to eat something special,
safely eating at a certain place)

Where I Am Now (somewhere in the middle)
Is there a milestone you've reached or
accomplishment you've made?
(Cleared for "may contain,"
ate/drank your allergen as a dose)

My Steps Up the Ladder
Things you've already done that have
helped you get closer to your goal
(started immunotherapy,
completed allergy testing,
did a food challenge,
took a medicine you needed)

Bottom Step (Where I started):
This may be one of the reasons you started
immunotherapy, including things you
wanted to do but couldn't, were afraid to
do, or felt like you were missing out on.

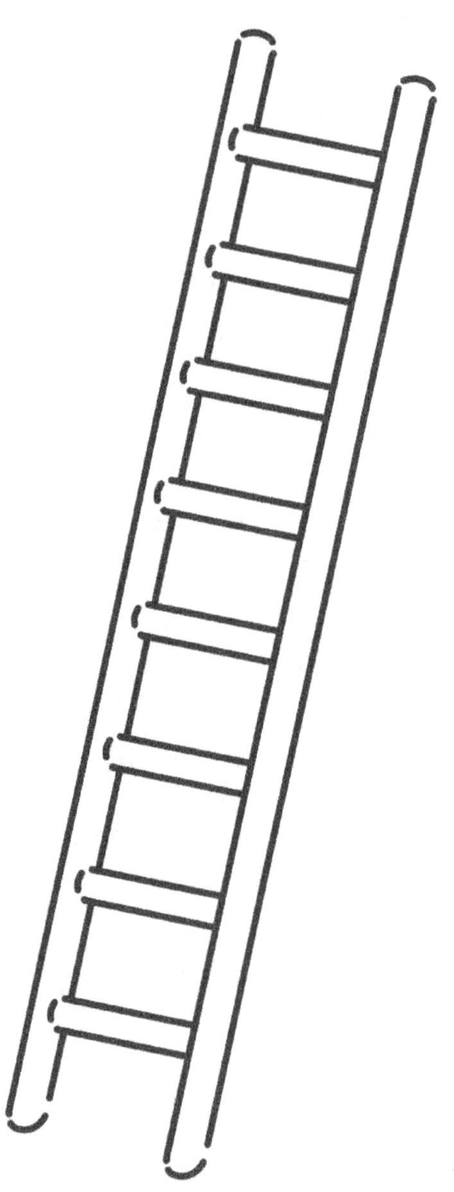

Look How Far You've Come!

Draw or write something you did that was really brave:

Draw or write something that used to feel scary but feels easier now:

Something I'm proud of:

When Things Feel Hard Again

Sometimes we forget how strong we are.

If things feel hard today or another time in the future, I can remind myself:
"I've already climbed this far."

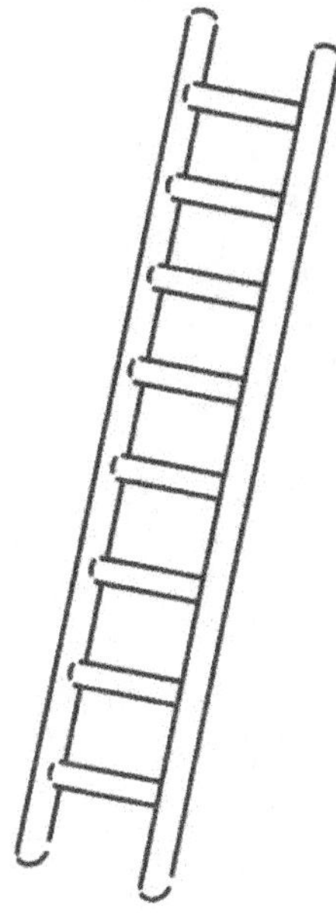

Redefining Success Beyond the Elimination of Risk

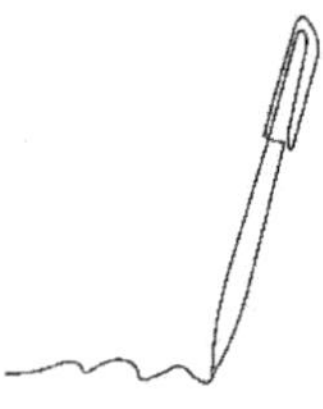

Initially, immunotherapy success is often defined by clear medical goals like reaching maintenance or protection from accidental exposure. Along the way, many notice meaningful changes they didn't expect, like increased confidence, flexibility, or reduced fear. These shifts can be easy to overlook because they happen gradually. This activity invites you to pause and recognize that progress.

Reflection Questions:

How did you originally define success in treatment?

How is that definition changing over time?

What small shifts have mattered more than you expected?

What forms of safety are present now that were not before?

What would it mean to measure success by quality of life, not just medical milestones?

Reducing fear, increasing trust, and expanding capacity are meaningful outcomes, even when risk still exists.

Part VII:
Arriving

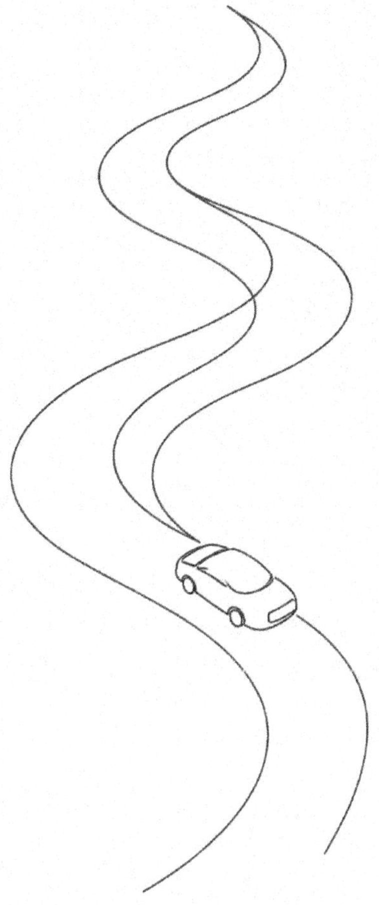

I can be changed by what happens to me.
I refuse to be reduced by it.

— Maya Angelou

Chapter 14:
Maintenance Phase

Maintenance, Setbacks, and Starting Again

Reaching maintenance was predictable, familiar, and manageable. We finished treatment just before the start of the COVID pandemic, so life opened up in new ways just as it shut down in many others. We had been excited to exist in the world with more ease, but restaurants, public events, and gatherings were on hold. We worked so hard for this freedom, and now there was nowhere to go with it.

There was a strange dissonance and yet a familiarity in pandemic life. While the rest of the world was adjusting, in many ways we felt uniquely prepared for the pandemic. Years of allergy management had already trained us in habits that became universal overnight: careful handwashing, cooking and meal planning at home, and having to consciously consider and create safety in daily activities.

This period also overlapped with one of the most difficult times in my personal life. My brother died in January 2020, and my own health challenges emerged in the months that followed. My son's "graduation" from peanut OIT was meant to be a celebration. Our whole family of five planned to join him for his final appointment where he would eat Reese's peanut butter cups for his dose, marking the transition into maintenance and giving him the flexibility to dose with peanut butter or another peanut candy he might enjoy. Life reshaped the moment, and the travel for the appointment had to be incorporated into the longer trip for my brother's memorial service. We tried to separate the emotional weight of the two events for the sake of the kids, but of course we were all feeling complicated emotions throughout that time. Fittingly, he didn't even like the Reese's.

We found our new rhythm easily at home, though. My son created his daily "trail mix" for his dose, a bowl of his maintenance peanuts and cashews with chocolate chips, raisins, and anything else he felt like adding. His brothers had their own versions too, and we always used separate bowls for theirs to visually and mentally distinguish his "dose" from their "snacks." It was shocking at first and healing over time to watch them all eat foods that were once dangerous.

Maintenance went smoothly for a long time, but a couple years in he started having occasional mild reactions. They were inconsistent and mostly mild, and the doctor looked to other explanations such as his dust allergy. This was one of the most difficult stretches of our journey. A mild but unexplained reaction was upsetting in a different way than one that was severe yet clear. My mind searched for explanations and solutions as we began logging food, completing breathing assessments to rule out asthma, and making changes at home to reduce dust. I tried to identify patterns and wondered if his braces might be a factor, since they were placed around the same time the reactions began and the symptoms often appeared around the time of his orthodontic appointments. I suspected a latex allergy or irritation from sores in his mouth after the orthodontic work.

It was emotionally exhausting to move back into problem-solving mode after feeling we'd found and achieved the "solution." It was also disheartening to feel restricted and worried again after experiencing that sense of freedom we'd found.

Eventually, additional testing revealed allergies to sesame and walnut. He'd eaten sesame as a toddler but tests were slightly high, and we had gotten conflicting information on whether to avoid or incorporate it into the diet. He'd passed a pecan challenge and the next step planned was an in-office challenge for walnut, but it was delayed due to the pandemic. I blamed myself for not pushing for clearer answers and letting these things that seemed like less of a priority fall to the side. I could understand rationally that this was not a failure and that I had been navigating an extraordinary amount. I knew that my son was so much safer now thanks to his tolerance for peanuts and cashews through OIT. Emotionally, it felt like I had let him down.

At this point, my son was around twelve years old. The idea of beginning another round of OIT felt overwhelming for him. Treatment was now available locally, which would eliminate the eight hours of driving that our appointments used to require. However, the new routine would include multiple doses and post-dose rest periods to separate the old and new allergens being treated, and my son was not open to that. The very idea made him want to quit taking even his maintenance dose.

We talked through the options together and he made it very clear that he didn't need or want full incorporation of these foods into his diet. He just wanted protection from accidental exposure. He chose SLIT to treat these "new" allergens, and we dove back into treatment.

The process was easier and gentler. He progressed smoothly and quickly, we did our updoses virtually and had his SLIT solution mailed to us, and he reached maintenance without significant issues aside from what he called the "stupid tongue itch" early on. This is common with SLIT and resolved over time. Our doctor helped us simplify the process even further by transitioning him from expensive extracts to a real-food preparation we could make at home.

Despite the bumps, the detours, and the moments of doubt, my son's life is wider, freer, and more flexible than it was before. At times he has expressed frustration and anger about the complexity of his path, and he is also thankful for the treatment and the protection it has given him.

When the road became unclear, it was tempting to turn back. Our hope is that by moving forward instead, his treatments will allow him to choose his own path toward the full, busy life that awaits him.

When Safety Changes, Feelings Catch Up (With Relief Comes Grief)

For many families, passing a food challenge or removing an allergen from the "unsafe" list is expected to feel like pure relief. And often, there *is* relief. But alongside it, parents are frequently surprised by waves of emotion they did not anticipate: uneasiness, tenderness, tears, a sense of being off-balance, even fear despite knowing that the food is now considered safe.

This reaction is common in the experiences of those who have gone through the process. It can be confusing and even isolating to feel unsettled after receiving good news. Some parents wonder if something is wrong with them, or worry that their reaction means they do not truly trust the outcome. Others feel guilty for struggling when they believe they should be celebrating.

The nervous system prefers familiarity

Nothing about this response means you are weak, ungrateful, or overly anxious. It means your nervous system is doing exactly what it was designed to do. Its primary job is to keep you alive, not evaluate facts. It learns through experience, repetition, and pattern. For years, your body learned a very specific set of rules about what kept you/your child safe: avoid this food, check labels, ask questions, be alert, be ready.

When a food challenge is passed, the rules change. Even when the change is positive, the body often reacts with uncertainty. Familiar danger can feel safer than unfamiliar safety. The brain may understand that the risk has shifted, but the nervous system needs time and experience to update its expectations.

Recalibration

Passing a challenge is not just about adding a food back in. It is about removing a long-standing safety protocol. That can feel surprisingly vulnerable.

Think about how your body feels after a long period of stress. Even when the emergency is over, it takes time to come down. Muscles stay tight. Sleep may be disrupted. Emotions surface once there is room for them.

In the same way, your nervous system needs repeated experiences of safety before it can fully relax. One successful challenge or updose does not instantly undo years of learning. Recalibration happens gradually, through time and repetition.

Mixed Emotions

Relief and grief often arrive at the same time. Many people feel a sense of relief that the burden has become lighter, while also experiencing grief for the years of fear, effort, and adaptation it took to reach this point. There may also be grief for what was lost along the way, including missed experiences, constant vigilance, and the version of parenting or living you did not get to have. Feeling multiple emotions at once does not mean you are stuck in the past. It reflects that this transition is meaningful and worthy of acknowledgment.

Identity Shifts

For many patients and parents, food allergy management becomes woven into their identity, shaping daily routines, decisions, relationships, and their sense of self-trust. When that role begins to change, even for positive reasons, it can leave behind a quiet and often unexpected question about who they are now within this new phase. There may be uncertainty about what to do with the time, energy, and vigilance that once went toward constant protection. This transition can feel emotional, tender, and disorienting at first. In most cases, these feelings gradually settle as a new sense of normal begins to take shape.

The Body Learns Through Experience, Not Logic

Reassurance can be helpful, but it is not what updates the nervous system. The body learns safety through lived experience rather than through information alone. Each neutral or positive interaction with a previously feared food, each uneventful meal, and each moment where nothing harmful occurs contributes to this learning process. Over time, these repeated experiences help the nervous system recognize that the meaning of the food has changed. This is why patience with yourself is so important during this phase. You are not behind in your adjustment; you are actively learning in the way the body is designed to learn.

Joy Can Coexist with Vulnerability

It is common for joy and vulnerability to exist side by side during periods of transition. Feeling tender does not diminish gratitude, and feeling cautious does not mean that trust is not developing. These emotional layers often reflect the significance of what you have been through and what is changing. During this time, your nervous system is reorganizing around a new reality, and that process can take time. Approaching yourself with gentleness and understanding allows both the progress and the complexity of your experience to be honored.

When the Rules Change

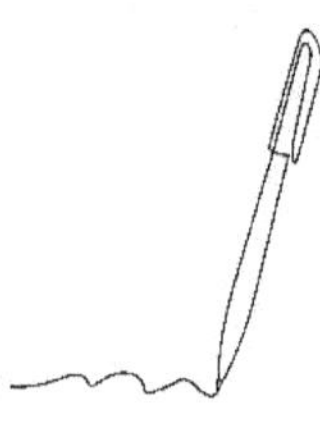

This page helps you notice how your body and emotions respond to positive change, especially when safety rules shift.

1. When I received good news about my/my child's allergy or challenge, I noticed these emotions:

____
____
____
____

2. In my body, I noticed:

☐ Tightness

☐ Restlessness

☐ Tearfulness

☐ Fatigue

☐ Alertness

☐ Relief

☐ Loosening

☐ Fluttering

☐ Other:

____
____
____
____

3. Thoughts that showed up included:

____
____
____
____

4. Protective habits that are still lingering for me:

____
____
____
____

5. What feels unfamiliar or tender about this new phase?

____

____

____

____

6. What might my nervous system need more of right now as it recalibrates?

☐ Time

☐ Repetition

☐ Reassurance

☐ Support

☐ Rest

☐ Permission to feel mixed emotions

7. Gentle reframe

Complete one or two sentences:

- "This reaction makes sense because…"

____

____

- "I can let this take time because…"

____

____

Chapter 15:
How The Journey Changes Us

Identity Shifts

 As treatment progresses and safety increases, many families expect that relief will naturally follow. Sometimes it does. Often, the internal sense of identity does not shift as quickly as the medical reality.

For years, you may have known yourself or your child in a very specific way. You were careful, vigilant, the one who brings the best safe cupcakes, the one who asks the questions. Much of the way you interacted with the world was based on creating and establishing safety. These are protective adaptations that developed over time, not just labels.

When treatment begins to change what is possible, those roles do not simply disappear. Instead, the change can feel unsettling. You may find yourself wondering: *If this is safer now, why does it still feel dangerous? If we let go of these routines, what keeps us safe?*

This is the discomfort of integration. When long-standing patterns begin to shift, even in positive ways, there can be a period of disorientation. This is especially true when the previous identity was built around safety and protection.

For some, this shows up as hesitation to take new steps, even when medically cleared. For others, it shows up as a pull to return to old routines that feel familiar. There may also be unexpected emotions such as grief, even as progress is being made.

Identity is not replaced all at once. It expands. You are not losing the parts of yourself that kept you or your child safe. You are learning how to carry them forward in a way that makes room for new experiences, new possibilities, and a different relationship with risk. That process takes time.

Just as your body and your child's body are adjusting to treatment, your internal sense of who you are in this experience is adjusting too. As you continue through this process, you may begin to notice that progress is not only about what your body can tolerate, but also about how your sense of safety, identity, and possibility slowly evolve alongside it.

Who We Were, Who We Are Becoming

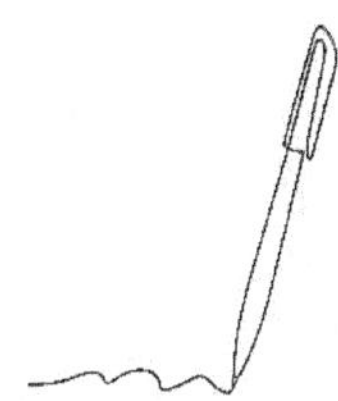

<table>
<tr>
<td>

Before Treatment
Describe yourself in relation to food allergies. What roles did you take on? What felt essential or central in life? What emotions were prominent?

</td>
<td>

Now
What has changed
What feels different (even if it is small)?
What feels possible or important now?

</td>
</tr>
<tr>
<td>

What Stays
What safety practices are still important?
What values remain the same?
What aspects of self are still central?

</td>
<td>

What Can Shift
What feels ready to change or soften?
What might you explore?
What aspects of self are shifting?

</td>
</tr>
</table>

My Allergy Journey Book: Telling Your Story in Your Own Way

This activity is based on a narrative therapy approach, which helps children make sense of their experiences by turning them into a story. When children can "see" their story, it becomes something they can understand, organize, and feel more in control of.

There is no right or wrong way to do this. The goal is not to create a perfect story, but to give your child a way to express their experience in a way that feels natural to them.

How to Begin

"We've been through a lot with your allergies and treatment. Sometimes it helps to tell the story of what we've been through. Do you want to make a book about your journey?"

If your child is unsure, you can start together and see what happens. Follow their lead.

Creating the "Book" (Keep It Simple)

You can make this as simple or as creative as your child would like:

- Staple a few pieces of paper together

- Fold paper in half to create pages

- Use a notebook or journal

- Create pages digitally if they prefer and print once complete

Let your child decide:

- Do they want to draw, write, or both?

- Do they want you to write the words for them?

- Do they want to tell the story out loud while you listen?

For younger children:

- They can draw pictures and dictate the story to you

- They can simply draw and give each page a title or a word

- Even a few pages is helpful

Story Prompts

Use sparingly and as needed, not all at once. Offer one at a time and follow your child's interest and attention. Begin with open ended questions ("What was it like?") and then incorporate their language into follow-up questions (If they say it was scary, ask what was scary).

Beginning the Story: What was it like before treatment?, What did you have to be careful about?

Starting the Journey: What was the first day like?, Was there anything that felt new?

The Middle of the Story: What were some hard moments?, What helped you get through them?

Moments of Change: When did things start to feel different?, Was there a moment you felt proud?

Now: What is life like now?, What feels easier or different?

Looking Ahead: What do you hope happens next?, What will it be like in 5 years? 10 years?

Adding Meaning to the Story: If it feels natural, you can gently highlight themes (bravery, practice, learning, teamwork, growth). You might say: "I notice you kept going even when it was hard" to help children see themselves from an outside perspective.

Optional Creative Elements: If your child is interested, they can:

- Give themselves a character name
- Add "helpers" (doctor, parent, sibling, stuffed animal)
- Draw "obstacles" and how they got past them
- Create a cover page with a title
- Revisit the book later and add new pages

Supporting the Process

Let your child lead the pace. Avoid correcting or reshaping their story. Focus on listening more than guiding. Validate their experience, even if it surprises you.

If your child only wants to draw, only wants to talk, or loses interest quickly, that is enough. The value is in the expression, not the finished product.

Closing the Activity

When your child is finished (for now), you might say:

"Thank you for sharing your story with me. I can see how much you've been through."

You can also ask:
"Do you want to keep adding to this later?"

This reinforces that their story is still unfolding.

Caregiver Reflection

- What did I learn about how my child sees this experience?
- Did anything surprise me?
- How can I support the story they are telling about themselves?

Maintaining Maintenance

 For many families, maintenance is imagined as the finish line. The part where the fear finally fades, the vigilance relaxes, and life simply becomes lighter, easier, and more "normal" again. Sometimes that happens. For others, maintenance asks for something quieter and more complex: adjustment.

For most patients, the intensity of OIT does recede as appointments and updoses are complete. But the adherence to a safety plan, rest periods, regular dosing (though perhaps not daily) and epinephrine carrying remain for most. The long-term routine will vary depending on the treatment or combination of treatments chosen. It will likely be less busy, stressful, and rigid, but will still require time and attention. Maintenance is not where effort and caution disappear. It is where effort becomes more subtle, more individualized, and more integrated into daily life.

Maintenance in the Real World

Maintenance means finding a way to merge the long-term routine into daily schedules, activities and events, late nights, vacations, holidays, and the social realities of life. This can be unsettling at first. Many patients and parents notice that their anxiety actually *spikes* during this phase because the structure that once ensured safety has loosened. You may find yourself mentally rehearsing scenarios again: What if dosing is late? What if we forget to mark down skip days? What if something feels off when we're away from home? This does not mean maintenance is failing. It means it is becoming real.

The goal is flexibility with intention and awareness. It is important to continue working with your allergist to understand what matters most, where there is room to adapt, and how to create routines that travel with you rather than tether you.

Shifting Responsibility

Maintenance also brings a developmental shift that can feel emotionally loaded: responsibility begins to move. Children who were once passive participants now become more active. Eventually, allergy management and the dosing routine becomes their responsibility. For many parents, this transition is both hopeful and terrifying.

Looking ahead toward the long-term goal can be helpful in gradually transferring skills, confidence, and trust in a way that matches your child's readiness over time. This process is rarely linear. There may be steps forward and steps back, especially during periods of stress, illness, or major life transitions. What matters most is that responsibility is shared before it is handed over completely. Maintenance is a long runway for practicing this together.

When Maintenance Feels Shaky

There might be moments in maintenance when confidence wobbles. A stomach bug might cause a long pause in dosing. Doses may be missed or symptoms may return. Old fears may resurface and a child who willingly dosed may become resistant again. These moments can feel discouraging, especially because it is natural to hope that maintenance means you were past these old hurdles.

Setbacks or regressions during maintenance are not failures. Often, what helps most is returning to the basics: clear plans, predictable routines, collaboration with your care team, and reassurance rooted in what you already know and have probably already successfully navigated.

Language and Expectations

One of the most delicate parts of maintenance is language. Words like *cured*, *fixed*, or *done* can feel tempting, especially after years of vigilance. They can also set families up for unnecessary disappointment or fear when normal fluctuations occur. Different treatments and providers may use different language to describe this phase. Regardless of phrasing, maintenance does not usually mean the complete absence of allergy and any consideration of it. It is a different relationship with it.

Using language like *protected*, *desensitized*, or *maintained* allows space for both hope and realism. It honors the progress that has been made without suggesting that attention is no longer required. Even for those who achieve "free eating" or "remission" may be advised to continue carrying epinephrine and/or to eat the allergen consistently.

Overpromising can make future challenges feel like betrayal or failure. Grounded optimism, on the other hand, builds resilience. Maintenance may feel quieter, but it asks for intention, especially at first. It requires recalibrating routines, redefining safety, and learning when to step back and when to lean in. There may be moments when you miss the structure of early treatment, even as you're grateful to be past it. That is normal.

Over time, maintenance becomes less something you *do* and more something you *live*. Confidence grows not because nothing ever happens, but because you learn, again and again, that you can handle what does. In the end, that may be one of the most meaningful outcomes of all.

Continuing the Journey

Reaching maintenance in immunotherapy can feel like arriving at a long-awaited destination. But maintenance does not mean the journey is over, it means the direction of travel may change.

During the early stages of treatment, energy is spent moving toward a specific goal. Whatever the destination looked like, treatment often provides a clear direction to move in. When maintenance begins, something shifts. The road no longer points only toward treatment milestones. Instead, the path begins to open outward toward the rest of life.

For some, this might mean expanding food choices, social experiences, or travel. Anxiety may soften as confidence grows. At times it may feel like you are moving quickly away from the place where the allergy once defined so much of daily life. At other times, the pace may slow. Some families move more gradually as they rebuild trust with foods, restaurants, schools, or social events. Sometimes we pause along the road to process the emotions that were pushed aside while focusing on the logistics of treatment. And occasionally, we may even take a few steps backward for a while for mental, social, or medical reasons.

All of this is part of the journey. Wherever the road leads, the experiences that brought you here do not disappear. The allergy experiences we have lived through, and the places we traveled in order to manage them, shape us in lasting ways.

Sometimes those places begin to fade into the distance as life expands. They may continued to impact how we think, understand ourselves, and how we interact with the world.

Even if life begins to look very different, we carry forward the skills we developed along the way. We remember the resilience we built. We bring with us the ways we learned to advocate, to problem solve, to adapt, and to care for ourselves and one another. Those parts of the journey come with us wherever we go next.

Moving the Goalposts

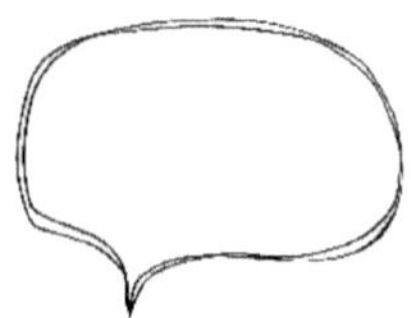

For a long time, maintenance lived in my mind as a finish line. After we crossed it, things would finally settle. I imagined a version of life where the rules stopped changing, where the constant recalibration was no longer necessary, and where I could exhale in a way I had not been able to before.

I pictured ordinary moments feeling easy again. Walking into a store without scanning, saying yes to things without mentally running through every possible outcome, trusting that we had finally arrived somewhere steady. While all this is true, I also learned that maintenance is not a destination. It is a different and complex relationship with uncertainty.

This phase is far quieter than the early days of treatment. There are fewer clinic visits, fewer adjustments, and much less intensity woven into our daily routines. Almost every aspect of life has become easier. Shopping, cooking, eating out, socializing, traveling, and even navigating my son's growing independence now feel more flexible and less burdensome. We can pick up and go when we want to. We can be more spontaneous. We can sit down at a restaurant without the same level of vigilance that once accompanied every decision.

We also discovered something unexpected. We are not actually a family that thrives on constant spontaneity or last-minute plans. We enjoy them occasionally, but we tend to prefer slower, more intentional rhythms. We like cooking at home. We like knowing what to expect and we enjoy our cozy routines. It is impossible to know how much of that was shaped by our allergy experience and how much is simply who we are, but it no longer feels important to separate the two. What matters is that we do not feel limited. The choice is ours now. We are not restricted from participating in life. We are choosing the version of it that fits us best.

For my son, that new freedom shows up in small ways that matter to him. He enjoys being able to eat a wider range of foods, including things with "may contain" labels that were once completely off limits. He can have snacks with friends more easily and naturally. He can move through social spaces with less explanation and less caution, which allows him to be more himself and less "allergy kid." These are small things on the surface, but they carry a kind of ease that was not always available to him.

As my son has grown, maintenance has also brought a gradual shift in responsibility. His awareness of his body and his role in his own safety have deepened over time. That awareness is both empowering and, at times, heavy. There is a particular weight that comes with knowing you are responsible for something important, especially when that something is your own health and safety. I've been careful not to hand it over all at once, but to guide him, support him, and allow him to step into it in ways that feel manageable.

What has surprised me most about this phase is that the most meaningful changes are not just about food, logistics, or even safety. They are about who we have become. My confidence as a mother is stronger and more grounded than I could have imagined at the beginning of this journey. My ability to trust my instincts, to advocate, and to care for my children in complex and high stakes situations feels deeply rooted now. Our connection as a family has been shaped by everything we have moved through together. There is a closeness, a shared understanding, a trust, and a sense of resilience that was built mostly through moments that felt difficult while we were in them.

My son carries this experience with him, too. He knows what it feels like to set his mind to a deeply meaningful task and accomplish it. He has taken care of himself. He has faced fear and continued forward. He has developed values and awareness that many people have no reason to develop so early in life. There is a depth of connection that forms when you navigate something hard together over time. In that way, we are deeply connected and trusting of one another, and that is the outcome that I am most grateful for.

Reflection Activity: Looking Back at the Road Traveled

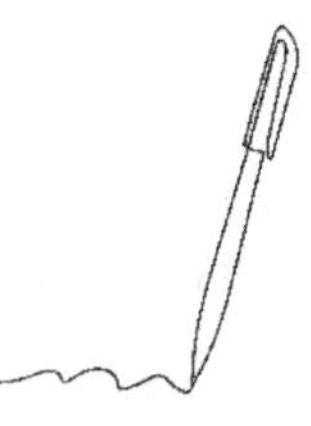

Every journey leaves some things behind and carries other things forward. This activity is an opportunity to reflect on the road you have traveled and the strengths you developed along the way.

Think about the beginning of your allergy journey.

What did life look like then?

____

____

What were some of the hardest parts of that time?

____

____

Now think about the journey through treatment.

What challenges did you work through?

____

____

What strengths or skills did you develop along the way? (Examples might include advocating for yourself, staying calm during stressful moments, problem solving, or supporting one another)

____

____

Now imagine the road ahead.

What are some things you are excited to move toward as treatment becomes less central to everyday life?

____

____

Even as life moves forward, what parts of this journey do you want to carry with you?

____

____

Activity for Kids: The Map of My Journey

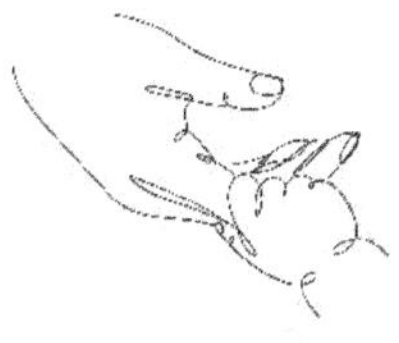

Imagine your allergy journey as a map with different places you have visited.

Draw or list some of the stops along your path.

Examples might include: learning about allergies, first reactions, starting treatment, brave moments, hard days, big wins, favorite memories, support from others, things you want to remember

Now think about the tools you picked up along the way.

These might be things like courage, patience, asking for help, or learning how your body works.

My Travel Tools:

Finally, think about where the road might go next.

What are you excited about doing as life continues to grow beyond treatment?

My Next Adventures:

Chapter 16:
How Far We've Traveled

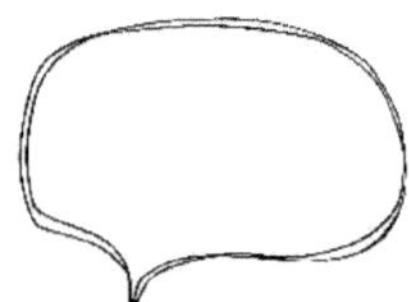

Sometimes I try to quantify it, even though there is no way to calculate just how far we've really come.

The numbers only tell a small part of the story, but by my best estimates, our journey has included:
about 30,000 miles driven,
over 700 hours in the car,
around 3,000 OIT doses and another 3,000 SLIT doses,
many thousands of dollars,
many tears shed,
countless labels read,
endless moments of advocating, explaining, double-checking,
and, if I'm honest, a handful of moments of second-guessing.

All of this effort was so that my son could arrive somewhere different. He has reached a place where previously life-threatening foods can now be safely tolerated. He lives with fewer moments of fear and doubt, and with more room for inclusion, connection, and ease.

But these numbers don't fully represent what this experience has meant. When I look back, I don't only see miles driven or doses completed. I see what filled those hours and distances. I remember the long drives where we found our favorite rest stops and the podcasts and music we shared along the way. I think about the books he read out loud to me while I drove and the conversations we had simply because we had the time and space to have them.

I also see a child who (I hope) knows that I would do anything for him, and that I am unwaveringly committed to his safety and well-being. Most meaningfully, I see the way we became more connected through this process. Our bond was strengthened because of the challenges, not in spite of them. That connection has become the most meaningful part of this journey for me, and it is something I would choose again without hesitation if he needed me to.

This is not a book about doing things perfectly. *Choosing treatment is not what makes a parent loving, committed, or devoted.* Choosing not to pursue treatment is absolutely not a lesser path, and requires just as much dedication, love, and devotion. Every path in this food allergy life demands so much from us. Every patient and family invests time, energy, emotion, and resources in ways that reflect their unique circumstances, values, access to care, and capacity.

All of these paths are real, and all of them are valid. Each one is an expression of care. Only you can determine what is best for you or your child in this moment and in the moments to come. My intention has simply been to share what our path has looked like to help you more clearly visualize your own.

If I could go back and speak to the version of myself who stood at the beginning of this journey, overwhelmed and searching while being told there were no options, I would tell her this:

You will find your way. Your path may not look like anyone else's, and it may not be straightforward. It may change as you move forward, but you will find a way.

I don't know how many miles you'll travel, how many decisions you will need to make, or how much time, energy, and resources your path will require. I can't tell you what direction you should choose. I can only hope that this book has helped you feel less alone at whatever point you are now on your own path. I hope it has provided you with information you can trust, space to reflect, and tools to support you along the way. Most of all, I hope it has reminded you that you do not need to have the entire route mapped out before you begin.

Sometimes the next step is simply choosing a direction and turning toward it. You can trust that even if the road winds, if you pause, or if you change course along the way, you are still moving forward. You are still finding your way.

Wherever you go from here, may you travel with greater clarity, more steadiness, and the sense that you are not navigating it alone.

The Road Ahead: A Closing Reflection

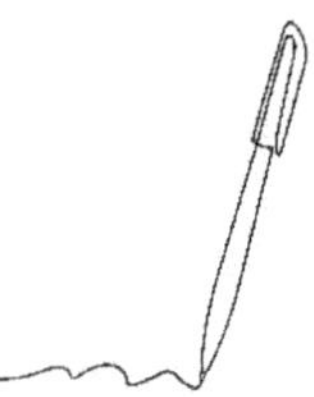 Your allergy journey has been a road with many twists and turns. You've traveled through moments that felt challenging, confusing, or even frightening. You've also discovered moments of bravery, resilience, and joy along the way. Every stop, twist, turn, and milestone has shaped who you are today.

Reaching this point in your journey does not mean the road ends. Instead, it opens up in new directions. Some paths may take you quickly away from what life used to look like. Others may loop back, asking you to revisit places you thought you had left behind. All of that is okay. Every step, whether forward, sideways, or backwards, is part of the adventure of learning, growing, and discovering what life can look like now.

The experiences you've had, the challenges you've faced, and the skills you've built are all part of your travel toolkit. You carry them with you like souvenirs from past trips: a reminder of what you've overcome and proof of the strength you've gained. Even when life changes, or new challenges appear, these tools will help guide your way.

Take a moment now to look back and look forward:

Look back: What are you proud of from your journey? What lessons or skills did you pick up along the way?

____

____

Look forward: What adventures are ahead? What do you hope to discover, explore, or try as you continue traveling your road?

____

____

Carry with you: What parts of your journey do you want to keep close, like tools in your backpack, that will help you along the way?

____

____

Remember: the journey is yours. You get to move at your own pace, explore new directions, and carry the best of what you've learned forward. And just like any traveler, you may sometimes rest, sometimes run, sometimes pause—but the road ahead is full of possibility.

No matter what comes next, you are prepared. You are capable. And you are never alone on this journey.

Your adventure continues.

My Allergy Adventure Map

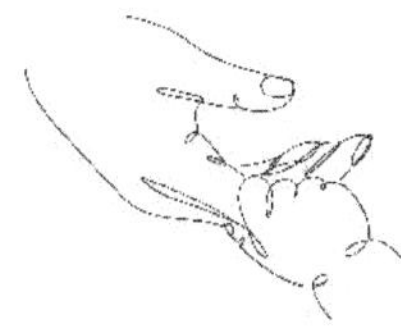 If your child used the map handout to track their progress through immunotherapy, use that for this activity. If you created a chart or log of your own, use this page as a guide to revisit that together.

Wow! Look at all the places you've traveled on your allergy adventure! You've faced tricky spots, learned new skills, and grown braver every step of the way. Now it's time to reflect on your journey and imagine the roads ahead.

Look Back: Draw or write about a stop on your map where you felt proud of yourself. What happened there? Draw a little picture of that part of your journey:

Look Forward: The road ahead is full of new adventures! What might you choose to explore next?

Tools in My Backpack: What superpowers, skills, or things you've learned along the way will help you on other adventures in the future?

References

Abramowitz, J. S., Deacon, B. J., & Whiteside, S. P. H. (2019). *Exposure therapy for anxiety: Principles and practice* (2nd ed.). Guilford Press.

Afzal, N., Ye, S., Page, A. C., Trickey, D., Lyttle, M. D., Hiller, R. M., & Halligan, S. L. (2022). A systematic literature review of the relationship between parenting responses and child post-traumatic stress symptoms. *European Journal of Psychotraumatology, 14*(1), 2156053. https://doi.org/10.1080/20008066.2022.2156053

American Psychiatric Association. (2022). *Diagnostic and statistical manual of mental disorders* (5th ed., text rev.; DSM-5-TR). American Psychiatric Publishing. https://doi.org/10.1176/appi.books.9780890425787

Anagnostou, K., Islam, S., King, Y., Foley, L., Pasea, L., Bond, S., Palmer, C., Deighton, J., Ewan, P., & Clark, A. (2014). Assessing the efficacy of oral immunotherapy for the desensitisation of peanut allergy in children (STOP II): A phase 2 randomised controlled trial. *The Lancet, 383*(9925), 1297–1304. https://doi.org/10.1016/S0140-6736(13)62301-6

Arasi, S., Otani, I. M., Klingbeil, E., Bégin, P., Kearney, C., Dominguez, T. L. R., Block, W. M., O'Riordan, G., & Nadeau, K. C. (2014). Two year effects of food allergen immunotherapy on quality of life in caregivers of children with food allergies. *Allergy, Asthma & Clinical Immunology, 10*(1), 57. https://doi.org/10.1186/1710-1492-10-57

Buckey, T. M., Frangiosa, J., Diem, L., Hanna, E., Datta, R., Gober, L., Brown-Whitehorn, T., Spergel, J. M., Muir, A., & Cianferoni, A. (2026). *Eosinophilic esophagitis incidence during single and multiple food oral immunotherapy*. Annals of Allergy, Asthma & Immunology. Advance online publication. https://doi.org/10.1016/j.anai.2026.02.007

Castellana, E., & Chiappetta, M. R. (2025). Sublingual immunotherapy: Insights into clinical benefits and safety profile. *Hospital Pharmacy*. Advance online publication. https://doi.org/10.1177/0018578725140299

Cordova, D. I., & Lepper, M. R. (1996). Intrinsic motivation and the process of learning. *Journal of Educational Psychology, 88*(4), 715–730. https://doi.org/10.1037/0022-0663.88.4.715

Craske, M. G., Treanor, M., Conway, C. C., Zbozinek, T., & Vervliet, B. (2014). Maximizing exposure therapy: An inhibitory learning approach. *Behaviour Research and Therapy, 58*, 10–23. https://doi.org/10.1016/j.brat.2014.04.006

Crespo, C., Santos, S., Canavarro, M. C., Kielpikowski, M., Pryor, J., & Féres-Carneiro, T. (2013). Family rituals and quality of life in pediatric chronic illness. *Journal of Family Psychology, 27*(3), 389–398. https://doi.org/10.1080/00207594.2013.806811

Deci, E. L., & Ryan, R. M. (1985). *Intrinsic motivation and self-determination in human behavior.* Plenum.

Dhami, S., Nurmatov, U., Arasi, S., Khan, T., Asaria, M., Zaman, H., Agarwal, A., Netuveli, G., Roberts, G., Pfaar, O., & Sheikh, A. (2017). Allergen immunotherapy for the treatment of allergic rhinitis and/or asthma: An umbrella review. *Allergy, Asthma & Clinical Immunology, 13*(1), 1–14. https://doi.org/10.1186/s13223-017-0209-1

Duncanson, E., Le Leu, R. K., Shanahan, L., Macauley, L., Bennett, P. N., Weichula, R., McDonald, S., Burke, A. L. J., Collins, K. L., Chur-Hansen, A., & Jesudason, S. (2021). The prevalence and evidence-based management of needle fear in adults with chronic disease: A scoping review. *PLoS ONE, 16*(6), e0253048. https://doi.org/10.1371/journal.pone.0253048

Feldman, R. (2007). Parent–infant synchrony: Biological foundations and developmental outcomes. *Current Directions in Psychological Science, 16*(6), 340–345. https://doi.org/10.1111/j.1467-8721.2007.00532.x

Fiese, B. H., & Everhart, R. S. (2006). Medical adherence and childhood chronic illness: Family daily management skills and emotional climate as emerging contributors. *Current Opinion in Pediatrics, 18*(5), 551–557. https://doi.org/10.1097/01.mop.0000245357.68207.9b

Fiese, B. H., Tomcho, T. J., Douglas, M., Josephs, K., Poltrock, S., & Baker, T. (2002). A review of 50 years of research on naturally occurring family routines and rituals: Cause for celebration? *Journal of Family Psychology, 16*(4), 381–390. https://doi.org/10.1037/0893-3200.16.4.381

Gentsch, A., & Kuehn, E. (2022). Clinical manifestations of body memories: The impact of past bodily experiences on mental health. *Brain Sciences, 12*(5), 594. https://doi.org/10.3390/brainsci12050594

Greenhawt, M., Albright, D., Anvari, S., Arends, N., Arkwright, P. D., Bégin, P., Blümchen, K., Brown-Whitehorn, T., Cassell, H., Chan, E. S., Ciaccio, C. E., Deschildre, A., Divaret-Chauveau, A., Dorris, S., Dorsey, M., Du Toit, G., Eiwegger, T., Erlewyn-Lajeunesse, M., Fleischer, D. M., et al. (2025). Efficacy and safety of epicutaneous immunotherapy in peanut-allergic toddlers: Open-label extension to EPITOPE. *Journal of Allergy and Clinical Immunology: In Practice, 13*(5), 1176–1187.e7. https://doi.org/10.1016/j.jaip.2025.02.004

Ho, S., Cooke, F., Ramos, A., McQuaid, E. L., Sharma, H., & Herbert, L. J. (2024). Anxiety among youth with food allergy. *Journal of Pediatric Psychology, 49*(7), 473–481. https://doi.org/10.1093/jpepsy/jsae026

Howe, L. C., Leibowitz, K. A., Perry, M. A., Bitler, J. M., Block, W., Kaptchuk, T. J., Nadeau, K. C., & Crum, A. J. (2019). Changing patient mindsets about non-life-threatening symptoms during oral immunotherapy: A randomized clinical trial. *The Journal of Allergy and Clinical Immunology: In Practice, 7*(5), 1550–1559. https://doi.org/10.1016/j.jaip.2019.01.022

Ilyasova, A. A., & Kim, E. H. (2026). Sublingual immunotherapy for food allergy: Updates in safety, efficacy, and future considerations. *Current Allergy and Asthma Reports, 26*(1), 1. https://doi.org/10.1007/s11882-025-01244-3

Iyengar, S. S., & Lepper, M. R. (2000). When choice is demotivating. *Journal of Personality and Social Psychology, 79*(6), 995–1006. https://doi.org/10.1037/0022-3514.79.6.995

Iyengar, S. S., Wells, R. E., & Schwartz, B. (2006). Doing better but feeling worse. *Psychological Science, 17*(2), 143–150. https://doi.org/10.1111/j.1467-9280.2006.01677.x

Keet, C. A., Frischmeyer-Guerrerio, P. A., Thyagarajan, A., Schroeder, J. T., Hamilton, R. G., Boden, S., Steele, P., Driggers, S., Burks, A. W., & Wood, R. A. (2012). The safety and efficacy of sublingual and oral immunotherapy for milk allergy. *Journal of Allergy and Clinical Immunology, 129*(2), 448–455. https://doi.org/10.1016/j.jaci.2011.10.023

Kim, E. H., & Burks, A. W. (2020). Sublingual immunotherapy for food allergy and its future directions. *Immunotherapy, 12*(12), 921–931. https://doi.org/10.2217/imt-2020-0123

Langer, E. J., & Rodin, J. (1976). The effects of choice and enhanced personal responsibility. *Journal of Personality and Social Psychology, 34*(2), 191–198.

https://doi.org/10.1037/0022-3514.34.2.191

Li, J.-B., Yang, A., Dou, K., & Cheung, R. Y. M. (2020). Self-control moderates the association between perceived severity of coronavirus disease 2019 (COVID-19) and mental health problems among the Chinese public. *International Journal of Environmental Research and Public Health, 17*(13), 4820. https://doi.org/10.3390/ijerph17134820

Lieberman, M. D., Eisenberger, N. I., Crockett, M. J., Tom, S. M., Pfeifer, J. H., & Way, B. M. (2007). Putting feelings into words: Affect labeling disrupts amygdala activity in response to affective stimuli. *Psychological Science, 18*(5), 421–428. https://doi.org/10.1111/j.1467-9280.2007.01916.x

Lucendo, A. J., Arias, A., & Tenias, J. M. (2014). Relation between eosinophilic esophagitis and oral immunotherapy for food allergy: A systematic review with meta-analysis. *Annals of Allergy, Asthma & Immunology, 113*(6), 624–629. https://doi.org/10.1016/j.anai.2014.08.004

Marsteller, N. L., Morphew, T. L., & Randhawa, I. S. (2021). Demographic, clinical and diagnostic correlation of almond allergy in a cohort of nut allergy patients. *Food and Agricultural Immunology, 32*(1), 460–470. https://doi.org/10.1080/09540105.2021.1955831

McMurtry, C. M., Taddio, A., Noel, M., Antony, M. M., Chambers, C. T., Asmundson, G. J. G., Pillai Riddell, R., Shah, V., MacDonald, N. E., Rogers, J., Bucci, L. M., Mousmanis, P., Lang, E., Halperin, S., Bowles, S., Halpert, C., Ipp, M., Rieder, M. J., Robson, K., Uleryk, E., Votta Bleeker, E., Dubey, V., Hanrahan, A., Lockett, D., & Scott, J. (2016). Exposure-based interventions for the management of individuals with high levels of needle fear across the lifespan: A clinical practice guideline and call for further research. *Cognitive Behaviour Therapy, 45*(3), 217–235. https://doi.org/10.1080/16506073.2016.1157204

Misuraca, R., Nixon, A. E., Miceli, S., Di Stefano, G., & Scaffidi Abbate, C. (2024). On the advantages and disadvantages of choice. *Frontiers in Psychology, 15*, 1290359. https://doi.org/10.3389/fpsyg.2024.1290359

Mondello, W. (2021, December 20). Girl with milk allergy dies of severe reaction related to desensitization. *Allergic Living.* https://www.allergicliving.com/2021/12/20/girl-with-milk-allergydies-of-severe-reaction-related-to-desensitization/

Nachshon, L., Schwarz, N, Tsviban, L., Levy, M.B., Goldberg, M.R., Epstein-Rigby, N, Katc, Y., & Elizur, A. (2021). Patient characteristics and risk factors for home epinephrine-treated reactions during oral immunotherapy for food allergy. *Journal of Allergy and Clinical Immunology: In Practice, 9*(1), 185–192.e3. doi: 10.1016/j.jaip.2020.07.034

Nurmatov, U., Devereux, G., Worth, A., Healy, L., & Sheikh, A. (2014). Effectiveness and safety of orally administered immunotherapy for food allergy: A systematic review and meta-analysis. *British Journal of Nutrition, 111*(1), 12–22. https://doi.org/10.1017/S0007114513002353

Patel, N., Vazquez-Ortiz, M., & Turner, P. J. (2019). Risk factors for adverse reactions during oral immunotherapy. *Current Treatment Options in Allergy, 6*(3), 164–174. https://doi.org/10.1007/s40521-019-00205-2

Plessis, A. A., Cameron, S. B., Invik, R., Hanna, M., Mack, D. P., & Cook, V. E. (2024). Real-world experience: A retrospective pediatric chart review to determine why patients and caregivers discontinue oral immunotherapy. *Allergy, Asthma & Clinical Immunology, 20*, 54. https://doi.org/10.1186/s13223-024-00912-9

Quintana Mariñez, M.G., Chakkera, M., Ravi, N., Ramaraju, R., Vats, A., Nair, A.R., Bandhu, A.K., Koirala, D., Pallapothy, M.R., & Khan, S. (2022). The other sibling : A systematic review of the mental health effects on a healthy sibling of a child with a chronic disease. *Cureus, 11,* 14(9). http://doi.org/10.7759/cureus.29042

Ramos, A., & Herbert, L. (2020). The role of exposure therapy in treating food allergy related anxiety. *The Journal of Allergy and Clinical Immunology, 145*(2, Suppl.), AB74. https://doi.org/10.1016/j.jaci.2019.12.123

Randhawa, I., & Marsteller, N. (2024). Long-term efficacy and safety of cow's milk anaphylaxis specific immunotherapy: Allergen unresponsiveness via the Tolerance Induction Program. *Journal of Allergy and Clinical Immunology: Global, 3*(3), 100285. https://doi.org/10.1016/j.jacig.2024.100285

Roberts, K., Meiser-Stedman, R., Brightwell, A., & Young, J. (2021). Parental anxiety and posttraumatic stress symptoms in pediatric food allergy. *Journal of Pediatric Psychology, 46*(6), 688–697. https://doi.org/10.1093/jpepsy/jsab012

Romantsik, O., Tosca, M. A., Zappettini, S., Calevo, M.G. (2018). Oral and sublingual immunotherapy for egg allergy. *Cochrane Database of Systematic Reviews, 2018*(4), CD010638. https://doi.org/10.1002/14651858.CD010638.pub3

Ryan, R. E., & Hill, S. (2024). Decision aids: Challenges for practice when we have confidence in effectiveness. *Cochrane Database of Systematic Reviews, 2024*(1), ED000164. https://doi.org/10.1002/14651858.ED000164

Salkovskis, P. M. (1991). The importance of behaviour in the maintenance of anxiety and panic: A cognitive account. *Behavioural Psychotherapy, 19*(1), 6–19. https://doi.org/10.1017/S0141347300011472

Sato, S., Nagakura, K.-I., Yanagida, N., & Ebisawa, M. (2025). Recent advances in oral immunotherapy for food allergies. *Clinical Reviews in Allergy & Immunology, 68*(1), 89. https://doi.org/10.1007/s12016-025-09108-4

Sindher, S. B., Nadeau, K. C., Chinthrajah, R. S., Leflein, J. G., Bégin, P., Ohayon, J. A., Ponda, P., Wambre, E., Liu, J., Khokhar, F. A., Akinlade, B., Maloney, J., Orengo, J. M., Hamilton, J. D., Kamal, M. A., Hooper, A. T., Patel, N., Patel, K., Laws, E., Mannent, L. P., & Radin, A. R. (2025). Efficacy and safety of dupilumab in children with peanut allergy: A multicenter, open-label, phase II study. *Allergy, 80*(1), 227–237. https://doi.org/10.1111/all.16404

Soller, L., Abrams, E. M., Carr, S., Kapur, S., Rex, G. A., Leo, S., Lidman, P. G., Yeung, J., Vander Leek, T. K., McHenry, M., Wong, T., Cook, V. E., Hildebrand, K. J., Gerstner, T. V., Mak, R., Lee, N. J., Cameron, S. B., & Chan, E. S. (2019). First real-world safety analysis of preschool peanut oral immunotherapy. *The Journal of Allergy and Clinical Immunology: In Practice, 7*(8), 2759–2767.e5. https://doi.org/10.1016/j.jaip.2019.04.010

Spagnola, M., & Fiese, B. H. (2007). Family routines and rituals: A context for development in the lives of young children. *Infants & Young Children, 20*(4), 284–299. https://doi.org/10.1097/01.IYC.0000290352.32170.5a

Swee, M. B., Klein, K., Murray, S., & Heimberg, R. G. (2023). A brief self-compassionate letter-writing intervention for individuals with high shame. *Mindfulness, 14*(4), 854–867. https://doi.org/10.1007/s12671-023-02097-5

Teicher, M. H., & Samson, J. A. (2016). Annual research review: Enduring neurobiological effects of childhood abuse and neglect. *Journal of Child Psychology and Psychiatry, 57*(3), 241–266. https://doi.org/10.1111/jcpp.12507

Theodorakakis, M., Machado, S., Andre, M., Hazi, A., Ongaro, Z., Pan, L., Yap, S., Shreffler, W., & Pistiner, M. (2024). Parental experience administering epinephrine for systemic reactions during infant and toddler oral food challenges. *The Journal of Allergy and Clinical Immunology: In Practice, 12*(10), 2838–2841.e1. https://doi.org/10.1016/j.jaip.2024.06.045

Tian, T., Li, Y., Yuan, G., & Jiang, W. (2025). Efficacy and safety of dupilumab in patients with moderate-to-severe atopic dermatitis and comorbid allergic rhinitis. *Frontiers in Medicine, 12*, 1556769. https://doi.org/10.3389/fmed.2025.1556769

Trevisonno, J., Venter, C., Pickett-Nairne, K., Bégin, P., Cameron, S. B., Chan, E. S., Cook, V. E., Factor, J. M., Groetch, M., Hanna, M. A., Jones, D. H., Wasserman, R. L., & Mack, D. P. (2024). Age-related food aversion and anxiety represent primary patient barriers to food oral immunotherapy. *The Journal of Allergy and Clinical Immunology: In Practice, 12*(7), 1809–1818.e3. https://doi.org/10.1016/j.jaip.2024.03.014

Vickery, B. P., Berglund, J. P., Burk, C. M., Fine, J. P., Kim, E. H., Kim, J. I., Keet, C. A., Kulis, M., Orgel, K. G., Guo, R., Steele, P. H., Virkud, Y. V., Ye, P., Wright, B. L., Wood, R. A., & Burks, A. W. (2017). Early oral immunotherapy in peanut-allergic preschool children is safe and highly effective. *Journal of Allergy and Clinical Immunology, 139*(1), 173–181.e8. https://doi.org/10.1016/j.jaci.2016.05.027

Vickery, B. P., Vereda, A., Casale, T. B., Beyer, K., du Toit, G., Hourihane, J. O., Jones, S. M., Shreffler, W. G., Marcantonio, A., Zawadzki, R., Sher, L., Carr, W. W., Fineman, S., Greos, L., Rachid, R., Ibáñez, M. D., Tilles, S., Assa'ad, A. H., Nilsson, C., … Burks, A. W. (2018). AR101 oral immunotherapy for peanut allergy. *New England Journal of Medicine, 379*(21),

1991–2001. https://doi.org/10.1056/NEJMoa1812856

Wang, J., Jones, S. M., Pongracic, J. A., Song, Y., Yang, N., Sicherer, S. H., Makhija, M. M., Robison, R. G., Moshier, E., Godbold, J., Sampson, H. A., & Li, X.-M. (2015). Safety, clinical, and immunologic efficacy of a Chinese herbal medicine (Food Allergy Herbal Formula-2) for food allergy. *The Journal of Allergy and Clinical Immunology, 136*(4), 962–970.e1. https://doi.org/10.1016/j.jaci.2015.04.029

Wang, W., Wang, X., Wang, H., & Wang, X. (2023). Evaluation of safety, efficacy, and compliance of intralymphatic immunotherapy for allergic rhinoconjunctivitis: A systematic review and meta-analysis. *International Archives of Allergy and Immunology, 184*(8), 754–766. https://doi.org/10.1159/000529025

Wasserman, R. L., Factor, J. M., Baker, J. W., Mansfield, L. E., Katz, Y., Hague, A. R., Paul, M. M., Sugerman, R. W., Lee, J. O., Lester, M. R., Mendelson, L. M., Nacshon, L., Levy, M. B., Goldberg, M. R., & Elizur, A. (2014). Oral immunotherapy for peanut allergy: Multipractice experience with epinephrine-treated reactions. *Journal of Allergy and Clinical Immunology: In Practice, 2*(1), 91–96. https://doi.org/10.1016/j.jaip.2013.10.001

Wei, C.-C., Lin, C.-L., Kao, C.-H., Liao, Y.-H., Shen, T.-C., Tsai, J.-D., Chang, Y.-J., & Li, T.-C. (2014). Increased risk of Kawasaki disease in children with common allergic diseases. *Annals of Epidemiology, 24*(5), 340–343. https://doi.org/10.1016/j.annepidem.2014.02.003

Whitehouse, A.R.D., & Chacko, T. (2026, June 9). Misconceptions, Myths & More: What Dr. Tom Chacko Wants You to Know About OIT (No. 79) [Audio podcast episode]. *Don't Feed the Fear.* https://www.buzzsprout.com/2371319/episodes/18695868

Whitehouse, A.R.D., & Chung, I. (2026, July 7). Choosing Not Now: Ina Chung on Involving Our Children in Treatment Decisions (No. 83) [Audio podcast episode]. *Don't Feed the Fear.* https://dontfeedthefear.buzzsprout.com

Whitehouse, A.R.D., & Danna, S. (2026, September 1). Setbacks, Symptoms, and Still Moving Forward: Sarah Danna's TIP Journey (No. 91) [Audio podcast episode]. *Don't Feed the Fear.* https://dontfeedthefear.buzzsprout.com

Whitehouse, A.R.D., & Fox, A. (2026, June 23). Mindset and Mental Health in OIT with Professor

Adam Fox (No. 81) [Audio podcast episode]. *Don't Feed the Fear.*
https://www.buzzsprout.com/2371319/episodes/18695868

Whitehouse, A.R.D., & Freeman, A. (2026, July 21). How Sublingual Immunotherapy Can Increase Safety and Freedom, With Dr. Allison Freeman (No. 85) [Audio podcast episode]. *Don't Feed The Fear.* https://www.buzzsprout.com/2371319/episodes/18807870

Whitehouse, A.R.D., & Grijalva, N. (2026, September 8). More Than We Expected: One Family's Journey Through Food Allergies, TIP, and Kawasaki (No. 92) [Audio Podcast Episode]. *Don't Feed the Fear.* https://dontfeedthefear.buzzsprout.com

Whitehouse, A.R.D., & Jones, D. (2026, June 2). From Controversy to Collaboration: The Evolution of OIT with Dr. Doug Jones (No. 78) [Audio podcast episode]. *Don't Feed the Fear.* https://www.buzzsprout.com/2371319/episodes/18690144

Whitehouse, A.R.D., & Li, X. (2026, September 9). Traditional Chinese Medicine: Dr. Xiu-Min Li's Groundbreaking Research (No. 95) [Audio podcast episode]. *Don't Feed the Fear.* https://www.buzzsprout.com/2371319/episodes/18839647

Whitehouse, A.R.D., & Mustafa, S. (2026, April 14). Shared Decision Making in Allergy Treatment Choices with Dr. Shazad Mustafa (No. 71) [Audio podcast episode]. *Don't Feed the Fear.* https://www.buzzsprout.com/2371319/episodes/18688026

Whitehouse, A.R.D., & Parrish, C. (2026, July 14). Demystifying EoE with Dr. Christopher Parrish (No. 84) [Audio podcast episode]. *Don't Feed the Fear.* https://www.buzzsprout.com/2371319/episodes/18820818

Whitehouse, A.R.D., & Randhawa, I. (2026, August 25). Understanding the Tolerance Induction Program (TIP) with Dr. Inderpal Randhawa (No. 90) [Audio podcast episode]. *Don't Feed the Fear.* https://www.buzzsprout.com/2371319/episodes/18784583

Whitehouse, A.R.D., & Relan, M.. (2026, April 28). Immunotherapy Options for Environmental Allergies with Dr. Manisha Relan (No. 73) [Audio podcast episode]. *Don't Feed the Fear.* https://www.buzzsprout.com/2371319/episodes/18687576

Whitehouse, A.R.D., & Schroeder, N. (2026, August 18). Is SLIT (Sublingual Immunotherapy)

Underrated? with Dr. Nikhila Schroeder (No. 89) [Audio podcast episode]. *Don't Feed the Fear*. https://www.buzzsprout.com/2371319/episodes/18807846

Whitehouse, A.R.D., & Stukus, D. (2026, April 21). Preparing for Immunotherapy: Dr. Dave Stukus on Tests, Challenges, and Expectations (No. 72) [Audio podcast episode]. *Don't Feed the Fear*. https://www.buzzsprout.com/2371319/episodes/18688026

Whitehouse, A.R.D., & Vickery, B. (2026, July 28). Biologics in Food Allergy Care: A New Era with Dr. Brian Vickery (No. 86) [Audio podcast episode]. *Don't Feed the Fear*. https://www.buzzsprout.com/2371319/episodes/18797430

Whitehouse, A.R.D., & Wada, K. (2026, August 4). Dr. Kara Wada on Sjögren's, ILIT, and Reimagining Immune Care (No. 87) [Audio podcast episode]. *Don't Feed the Fear*. https://www.buzzsprout.com/2371319/episodes/18797417

Wood, R. A., Togias, A., Sicherer, S. H., Shreffler, W. G., Kim, E. H., Jones, S. M., Leung, D. Y. M., Chinthrajah, R. S., et al. (2024). Omalizumab for the treatment of multiple food allergies. *New England Journal of Medicine, 390*(10), 889–899. https://doi.org/10.1056/NEJMoa2312382 Wang, J., Jones, S. M., Pongracic, J. A., Song, Y., Yang, N., Sicherer, S. H., Makhija, M. M.,

Yang, N., Wang, J., Liu, C., Song, Y., Zhang, S., Zi, J., Zhan, J., Masilamani, M., Cox, A., Nowak-Wegrzyn, A., Sampson, H., & Li, X.-M. (2014). Berberine and limonin suppress IgE production by human B cells and peripheral blood mononuclear cells from food-allergic patients. *Annals of Allergy, Asthma & Immunology, 113*(5), 556–564.e4. https://doi.org/10.1016/j.anai.2014.07.021

Yeung, J. P., Kloda, L. A., McDevitt, J., Ben-Shoshan, M., & Alizadehfar, M. (2012). Oral immunotherapy for milk allergy. *Cochrane Database of Systematic Reviews, 2012*(11), CD009542. https://doi.org/10.1002/14651858.CD009542.pub2

Zaazouee, M. S., Alwarraqi, A. G., Mohammed, Y. A., Badheeb, M. A., Farhat, A. M., Eleyan, M., Morad, A., Zeid, M. A.-A., Mohamed, A. S., AbuEl-Enien, H., Abdelalim, A., Elsnhory, A. B., Hrizat, Y. S. M. H., Altahir, N. T., Atef, D., Elshanbary, A. A., Alsharif, K. F., Alzahrani, K. J., Algahtani, M., Theyab, A., Hawsawi, Y. M., Aldarmahi, A. A., & Abdel-Daim, M. M.

(2022). Dupilumab efficacy and safety in patients with moderate to severe asthma: A systematic review and meta-analysis. *Frontiers in Pharmacology, 13*, 992731. https://doi.org/10.3389/fphar.2022.992731

Acknowledgments

No meaningful journey is ever taken alone, and this one is no exception.

This book was written in my mind during the long car rides to OIT appointments, late nights after tucking little boys into bed, and in the conversations with so many patients and parents who were carrying the same fears I once did. It was built from professional knowledge and lived experience on a foundation of the privilege of being trusted with other people's stories.

To the three best boys, thank you for being my reason for everything, including this book and all of my work. You were amazingly patient with my long writing stretches and distracted brain while I finished this project. You have taught me more about love, courage, flexibility, resilience, and perspective than any degree ever could. You have shown me that bravery usually looks very ordinary: taking a dose, asking a question, speaking up, trying again, and showing up anyway. Watching you navigate hard things has shaped the mother, the psychologist, and the person I have become. To CJ, Dad of the best three boys, thank you for standing in the middle of all of it with me, for taking my hand when things felt uncertain, and for helping me believe in myself and the work that I do.

A special thank you to Dr. Allison Freeman and Dr. Elizabeth Hawkins for generously spending your time reviewing the content of this book. Your support and expertise helped ensure that these pages were accurate and compassionate. I am sincerely grateful for your time, insights, support, and thoughtful feedback throughout this process.

Thank you to the following colleagues for your willingness to share your knowledge, time, and experience to make this book richer, wiser, and far more useful than I could have made it on my own: Dr. Doug Jones, Dr. Dave Stukus, Dr. Shahzad Mustafa, Dr. Farah Khan, Dr. Manisha Relan, Dr. Tom Chacko, Dr. Adam Fox, Dr. Christopher Parrish, Dr. Brian Vickery, Dr. Kara Wada, Dr. Nikhila Schroeder, Dr. Inderpal Randhawa, and Dr. Xiu-Min Li. Collaboration is a crucial part of this work, and I am deeply grateful for yours.

To my friends and guests who shared your stories, thank you for your honesty and openness: Mia Silverman, Natalie Grijalva, Sarah Danna, and Ina Chung.

And finally, to my clients, thank you for letting me walk beside you all these years. So much of what I know about healing has grown from you trusting me with your fear, your grief, your hope, your humor, your frustration, your strength, and your persistence. It has been an absolute honor to be a witness to your humanness.

About the Author

Amanda R. DeSio Whitehouse, PhD is a licensed psychologist specializing in anxiety, trauma, and nervous system regulation, with a clinical focus on supporting individuals and families navigating food allergies, celiac, and other chronic medical conditions. In addition to her clinical work, Dr. Whitehouse is the host of the *Don't Feed the Fear* podcast focusing on the social and emotional aspects of food allergy life. Her perspective is shaped not only by her professional training, but also by her personal experience as a parent navigating her own child's food allergies and various immunotherapy treatments. She is passionate about bridging the gap between medical care and emotional support so that patients and families feel informed, prepared, and supported throughout their own journeys.

In her therapy practice, Dr. Whitehouse combines her personal experience with her clinical expertise regarding somatic therapies and trauma-informed care into her unique approach to addressing the mental health needs of children, parents, and adults impacted by food-related medical needs. Her professional passions and certifications include trauma- and shame-informed care, somatic therapy for complex trauma, neurofeedback and other neuroscience-informed techniques, meditation instruction, and trauma-informed approaches to body image and emotional eating. Dr. Whitehouse also enjoys supporting the food allergy and celiac communities through speaking engagements, educational events, advocacy efforts, and professional trainings. She is available for booking by contacting Welcome@DrAmandaWhitehouse.com.

Outside her roles as a mom and psychologist, she can be usually be found enjoying her favorite forms of nervous system regulation: getting lost in books, spending time outdoors, and enjoying good music.

If This Workbook Helped You

If you found this workbook helpful, please consider leaving a review on Amazon to help other families find this resource. Reviews make a meaningful difference for small independent books like this, and your support is greatly appreciated!

You can follow my work at thefoodallergypsychologist.com and on Instagram and Facebook @thefoodallergypsychologist.

Sign up for my newsletter at thefoodallergypsychologist.com/connect/ to make sure you don't miss out on future offerings, including upcoming books already in progress.

The *Don't Feed The Fear* podcast is available on your favorite podcast platform and at DontFeedTheFear.buzzsprout.com.

Thank you so much for your support!

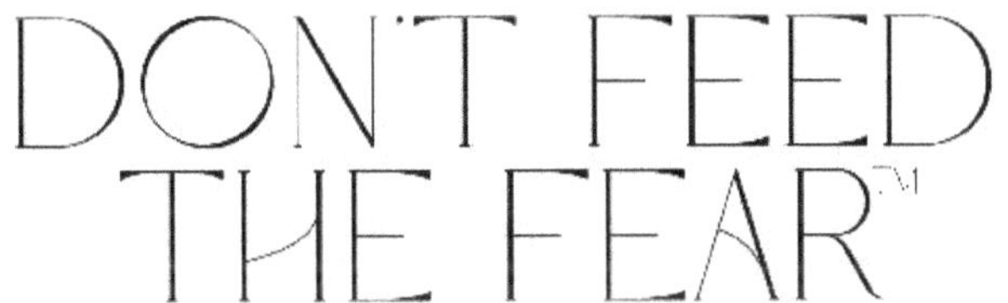

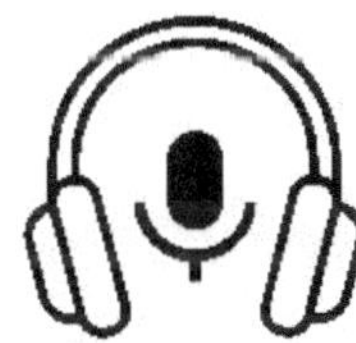